# I'M TOO YOUNG FOR THIS!

# I'M TOO YOUNG FOR THIS!

### The Natural Hormone Solution
### to Enjoy Perimenopause

## SUZANNE SOMERS

**HARMONY**

BOOKS · NEW YORK

The information in this book, including nutritional advice, hormonal or other therapeutic regimens, and all other information is the result of experience and research of the author, the persons interviewed for, or the other sources referenced in, this book. Not all of the information, statements, advice, opinions, or suggestions set forth in the interviews or material referenced or contained in this book have been evaluated by the FDA, and should not be relied upon to diagnose, treat, cure, or prevent any condition or disease. Before beginning any diet plan, exercise program, or therapeutic regimen, it is advisable to seek the advice of a physician. The author accepts no responsibility or liability for the use of any information or material contained in this book.

Copyright © 2013 by Suzanne Somers

All rights reserved.
Published in the United States by Harmony Books,
an imprint of the Crown Publishing Group,
a division of Random House LLC,
a Penguin Random House Company, New York.
www.crownpublishing.com

HARMONY BOOKS is a registered trademark of Random House LLC,
and the Circle colophon is a trademark of Random House LLC.

Originally published in hardcover in the United States by Harmony Books, an imprint of the Crown Publishing Group, a division of Random House LLC, New York, in 2013.

Library of Congress Cataloging-in-Publication Data
I'm too young for this!: the natural hormone solution to enjoy
perimenopause / Suzanne Somers.—First edition.
        pages cm
    1. Perimenopause—Hormone therapy—Popular works.
2. Progesterone—Therapeutic use—Popular works. 3. Middle-aged women—
Health and hygiene—Popular works.
    RG188.I48 2013
    618.1'75061—dc23          2013025638

ISBN 978-0-385-34771-6
eBook ISBN 978-0-385-34770-9

PRINTED IN THE UNITED STATES OF AMERICA

Design by Elizabeth Rendfleisch
Illustrations by Leslie Hamel
Cover design by Caroline Somers & Danielle Shapero-Rudolph
Cover photograph by Cindy Gold · Hair by Mooney

10  9  8  7  6  5  4  3  2

First Paperback Edition

*To Alan,*
*who hung in there*
*so we could live*
*happily ever after*

# CONTENTS

## ACKNOWLEDGMENTS

Heather Jackson, editor supreme at Crown, was my driver on this one. She has edited the last six books for me and always makes my books better. This one is no exception. Her keen sense of not overwhelming the reader as well as her strengths of eliminating redundancy and keeping the text on point (reminding me gently, and then sometimes not so gently, of the message of the book) all forced me to keep moving forward to make reading *I'm Too Young for This!* like an e-ticket on the expressway. As she says, this reader wants this information . . . now. Because Heather understood this she wouldn't let me linger. I tend to digress and go off in other directions that I feel you must know, but Heather kept saying "stay with the message." The reader wants to know how, what, and when. I like that Heather is that great combination of woman: sweet, smart, and strong. We are a great team. I thank you, Heather, for your excellence and your brain. You are a spectacular editor.

My thanks and gratitude to Dr. Prudence Hall for writing her insightful and knowledgeable foreword to this book. She is not only my friend but my trusted gynecologist. She has created the Hall Center in Venice, California, a cutting-edge medical space and place of serenity and beauty, making all who walk through her magnificent Indian-themed doors feel embraced and safe. You are immediately offered green or lemon balm tea, and while you sit and reflect you know you are in the right place. She is one of the very best in the field, a woman in menopause herself, therefore having a complete understanding of the passages that make women feel so out of their bodies. Women and men alike flock to her center.

Alan Hamel, my husband and partner in everything, shares absolute enthusiasm for all my projects and watches out for me in all arenas: legal, the deal, keeping away the wolves, and charming the prospects. He is a marketing genius, a true visionary, although he does have a tendency to overbook, but other than that, I am the luckiest woman on the planet to have a husband/manager who cares so deeply. He is the love of my life, a love deeply intimate and intertwined. We are both perfectly hormonally balanced, and because of that our life together is exciting, fun, and sexy.

Thanks to all who contributed their brain power, knowledge, expertise, and emotions. Women wrote me letters pouring their hearts out, begging for an answer. I was fueled by them because I knew I had the information to change their lives.

Dr. Jonathan Wright is always my go-to doctor for all answers regarding the new way to age. He uses "nature's tools" and was the first doctor in the United States to prescribe a full course of hormone replacement for women, offering them a quality of life never before achieved naturally. I appreciate his contributions once again.

Bill Faloon and his scientific staff graciously reviewed and provided feedback on the book while incorporating cutting-edge solutions for the perimenopause passage. Thanks to his brilliant scientific staff at the Life Extension Foundation, including: Dr. Luke Huber, Blake Gossard, April Roberts, Justin Henry, and

Dr. Scott Fogle. I am extremely grateful for my ongoing relationship with Bill Faloon and the Life Extension Foundation.

ForeverHealth.com will revolutionize this new type of care, making this approach for women and men accessible, affordable, convenient, and hopefully the next standard of care. Jim England, president of the Somers Companies has been instrumental in bringing Forever Health to fruition. I thank the initial team of outstanding doctors who share the Forever Health vision and joined the network: Dr. Michael Galitzer, Dr. Ron Rothenberg, Dr. Prudence Hall, Dr. Neil Rouzier, Dr. Theresa Ramsey, Dr. Rachel Burnett, Dr. Evelyn Brust, Dr. Larry Brock, Dr. Sean Breen, Dr. Joseph Upton, Dr. Cesar Lara, Dr. Sue Decotiis, Dr. Gail Gagnon, Dr. Anju Mathur, Dr. Joseph Raffaele, Dr. Gowri Rocco, and Dr. Marsha Nunley. Thanks to David Schmidt of LifeWave, Dr. Andy Jurow, my friend and nutrutionist supreme Brenda Watson, Dr. Rick Sponaugle, Dr. Bill Rae, and Dr. Ritchie Shoemaker for their contributions.

My design team once again gave me a great cover, under the direction of the EVP of our company, Caroline Somers, and Danielle Shapero-Rudolph. Caroline oversees the brand in all categories and always puts out beautiful, fresh-looking product with supersexy color and appeal. I've lost count of how many book covers we've done together, but I always love the most recent more than the last and I say that on every book. My thanks to both of you for always coming through with such perfection; and Caroline, I love you.

Once again, my daughter by marriage, Leslie Hamel, came through with her incredible talent and keen sense of humor in creating the illustrations of the Seven Dwarves of Perimenopause! She captured the combination of humor and frustration that defines this difficult passage. I knew she would nail it. Every dwarf makes me laugh or smile. Great work (as always). I love you.

And to my fabulous team at Crown: I adore our relationship, a real easy back-and-forth, all working together and never at odds, headed by our president and publisher, a strong and focused leader, Maya Mavjee, and Tina Constable, senior vice president and publisher of Crown Archetype. This is our twenty-first book together and it never gets old. Tina is a great person and a pleasure to work with. Thanks also to Mauro DiPreta, Tammy Blake, Meredith McGinnis, and Chris Tanigawa. Thanks to the sales group; I can't sell a book without them and they are the best: Christine Edwards, Andy Augusto, and Jacqui Lebow. And thanks to my copy editor, Laurie McGee. She was right there with me and I appreciate it.

Sandi Mendelson is my publicist extraordinaire, my maker of bestsellers, my taste authority, and my sexy girlfriend; I love working with her.

Cover photo by my go-to photographer, Cindy Gold, and her team, who make having pictures taken a breeze; and I love the look. Thanks to Bonnie Holland with her deft touch; thank you, Cindy and Bonnie, so much. And thanks to Mooney, who's been keeping my hair fabulous for the last twenty years and is such a pleasure to be with. We share a mutual passion for health and wellness.

Marc Chamlin is my attorney of many, many books. He knows the literary world, knows how to wade through the nuances of publishing nationally and internationally, and he keeps me happy and protected. He is still *the guy*!

Thanks to my friends at SexyForever.com.

To my fabulous "girls" who run the office: my great executive assistant, Julie Turkel, and my other fabulous personal assistant, Jordyn Goodman. Couldn't do it without you both.

Marsha Yanchuck, thanks for all the detail work and all our thirty-five years together. It's so appreciated.

And to my little friends, my cats, Betty and Gloria, who lie in my office window for hours, sleep on my chair, and come sit on my lap from time to time, keeping me company while I'm writing my books.

It does "take a village" and I am grateful for all who populate mine. Thanks all.

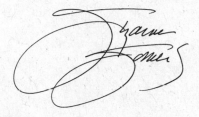

# FOREWORD

Do you remember when you woke up from a deep night's sleep and, like a child, bounded out of bed with energy and delight to greet a new day? When was the last time you looked in the mirror and felt beautiful and happy to be you? What about feeling madly in love and staying in bed all day with your beloved? Too many of my young patients in their thirties and early forties tell me it's been way too long since they've felt these youthful feelings. Instead, they tell me they're tired, gaining weight, depressed, angry, sleepless, and feeling just plain awful.

For the first few years of my medical practice, I thought these women sounded suspiciously menopausal, but their blood levels were almost always in the "normal" range. Well then, I thought, perhaps these patients were perimenopausal. During my ob-gyn residency at USC, perimenopause had been briefly mentioned as a woman's transition to menopause, usually beginning in her late forties or early fifties. I was taught it lasted about five or possibly ten years, but that it didn't require any specific medical treatment.

To gain insight on why my patients in their thirties and early forties felt so bad, I began testing their hormone levels, which I had never been taught to do. To my surprise, I started identifying subtle deficiencies in hormone levels in most of my young patients. I also started testing very young women on the birth control pill, and women who were postpartum. I found similar deficiencies. I realized these states were surprisingly similar to each other in terms of their symptoms and also in terms of their hormone levels. I had already been treating my menopausal patients for several years with bioidentical hormones, so I started treating these other conditions with them, too. To my surprise and happiness, these patients got well!

That was almost thirty years ago, and while my treatment of perimenopause has evolved and become more comprehensive, most doctors still don't recognize the existence of subtle perimenopausal changes. Because of that, often they won't check a young woman's hormones to establish healthy baselines, and they won't recommend treatment until a woman is well into menopause. A possible exception is the doctor who recommends the birth control pill as treatment for perimenopause. I feel treating perimenopause with the pill is terribly off base and is at best an ineffective Band-Aid. It usually makes women feel worse, due to suppressing their estrogen levels even more.

So what is my mainstay of perimenopausal treatment? I want to sing it out to the world and to every woman in need: bioidentical hormones are a woman's most effective therapy to help her experience vital health and youthful beauty. One of the most common causes of death in women is heart attacks. Bioidentical hormones also help prevent diabetes, high cholesterol, hypertension, and even deaths provoked by dementia in women.

Why don't women rush to balance their hormones back to youthful, healthy levels as soon as they begin to decline? They have heard there are no studies on bioidentical hormones to show their safety. They have been told hormones increase the risk of breast cancer and heart disease, and they are afraid. They are like a lot of doctors who have confused the data from synthetic nonbioidentical hormones (like Premarin and Provera) with bioidentical hormones. These are completely different hormones and do not react at all in the same way in the human body. In fact, bioidentical hormones have been studied extensively for the past seven or eight years. Here are a few of the studies documenting their safety:

- In 2007, the Mission Study followed 6,755 women for ten years and concluded that breast cancer was *not* increased in estrogen users (*see* Espié).
- In 1997, another study, published in the *Journal of Epidemiology*, followed 23,000 women who took bioidentical estradiol and bioidentical estriol, with and without progesterone. They had no increased risk of breast cancer. (*See* Schairer.)
- In 2007, a study was published that looked at 80,377 postmenopausal women who took bioidentical estradiol and progesterone; it showed no increase *or* decrease in breast cancer. Patients who took Premarin and Provera had a 69 percent increased risk of breast cancer. (*See* Fournier.)
- In 1996, the American Cancer Society published a study of 422,373 postmenopausal women who were cancer free at the beginning of the nine-year study. They found that women of all ages who took estrogens experienced a 16 percent decreased risk of dying from breast cancer, compared to nonusers, and that women who experienced natural menopause by the age of forty and who used BHRT had a 41 percent decreased chance of dying from breast cancer. (*See* Willis.)
- In 2008, a Japanese study published in the *International Journal of Clinical Oncology* looked at data from 5,861 patients from seven hospitals and concluded there was a

significantly negative correlation between estrogen use
and breast cancer (*see* Saeki).

- In 2008, data was published from 292 postmenopausal
  breast cancer patients who used BHRT. There was a 100
  percent survival rate among those patients who used BHRT
  for more than ten years. (*See* Christante.)

- In another study, 1,472 women with breast cancer who had
  positive estrogen receptors were followed by the University
  of South Wales. Their data, published in 2002, concluded
  that women taking estrogen and progesterone therapy had
  a 76 percent decrease in breast cancer reoccurrence, compared to nonestrogen users. (*See* Dew.)

- A study published in 2006 found that postmenopausal
  women with breast cancer had a decreased risk of mortality
  when using estrogen and progesterone hormone replacement therapy, compared to patients who didn't use estrogen after their breast cancer (*see* Batur). A study in 2004
  of perimenopausal women with breast cancer came to the
  same conclusions (*see* Durna).

So please, dear readers, please don't be afraid of these natural
bioidentical hormones. They perform all our body's functions,
like beating our heart, facilitating clear thoughts, cleansing toxins, and allowing normal growth and repair of our cells. We mistakenly believe our bodies can function without hormones. In
fact, if we suddenly lost all our hormones, we would die in less
than ten minutes.

Many of my patients question why we would want to interrupt
or change the natural course of our body's aging process. Why
would we want to interfere with our body's wisdom? Well, many
of our grandparents and parents didn't do so well aging naturally,
did they? They experienced a terrible loss of vitality and function. We don't have to live that way or decline as nature wills it.

It would be a rare individual who would turn down an antibiotic to save his or her life, yet that same person might decline a hormone that would prevent his or her death from a heart attack; both are "unnatural," yet wise decisions.

It basically comes down to this: the choices we make about our lives matter. The food we eat matters; how we exercise matters; our thoughts and the love we give and receive matters. Mark Whitwell's ThePromise.com helped me discover the importance of our choices; and the hormones and supplements we choose to replace or ignore, matter very much.

In your hands, you hold the secrets of all the right choices to make. Suzanne Somers offers yet again a groundbreaking contribution to the health and longevity of her readers with her comprehensive and extensive approach to perimenopause. With what gratitude I will recommend her book to my patients! I want them and you to be vital, beautiful, and healthy at every age, and to become, as the poet David Whyte encourages "the force that makes the river flow, and then the sea beyond." Let's all get on board and make this transition in life an illuminating ride to the joy and wisdom we all were created to share.

With love,
Prudence Hall, M.D.

The only constant is change. Learn to love it. As the rate of change accelerates, the result will appear chaotic to the uninitiated. But there is elegant order in chaos. Few so far have learned to recognize and profit from it. This is where the future lies.

—Frank Ogden

# INTRODUCTION

Is this you?

I had no idea what perimenopause was until a week ago! I'm pretty sure this is what is going on with my body! I'm a thirty-three-year-old having serious PMS symptoms, serious cramping, and all of a sudden a longer menstrual cycle. I'm also fatigued and I have gained ten pounds. I just made my annual and hope to get some answers!

—Melissa G.

I'm ten years on a roller-coaster ride of emotions. Hot flashes, night sweats. Yes, that would be me . . . Now the worst part is that my husband has just retired from the military. OMG! He hasn't lived at home in over a decade. He really doesn't know me and, wow, now I totally understand why couples break up at this age! It's so clear and so sad. I have no idea what is going to happen. All I can do is pray.

—Monique H.

I am going on about year five dealing with the loss of estrogen, progesterone, and other hormones that used to fuel me. I have experienced anxiety, loss of energy, and a loss of my zest for living.

—Andrea R.

I don't know who I'm living with anymore. Whether the real "me" will show up in the morning, or the bitchy, nasty person who I barely recognize as myself will arrive instead. I yell at my boys way too often. I'm cranky with my husband. I don't want to be around me when I'm like this, and frankly, I'm like this more than I'd like to be. It seems that when I was younger, I could count on PMS for the week before my period, and then life would return to normal. Now, it feels like if I get a "serene" week each month, that's the new normal.

My friends all say the same thing: we're too young for this. But what do we do about it? I grab for the chocolate to feel better or the needed glass of wine at the end of the day . . . or the chips and comfort crap and try to knuckle my way through it. Then I feel bad because when I grab for these crutches I'm not taking care of myself. What a crazy cycle!

I'm scared of being this shrewish, nasty shell of myself. But I'm also scared of drugs and hormone replacement. What are my options? I don't want to spend the next decade being in a bad mood. Life is too short to feel like this! It will ruin what should be fun years with my family and husband.

What are my/our choices? What can I eat, do, shift in my lifestyle to feel better? Forget about feeling better, how do I feel great? What do I avoid? I don't think I'm the only woman who is confused about whether to take hormones, which feel scary, or whether to leave be and try to address it by other means first. What's the latest research

say? Are there baby steps anyone can take to start moving in the right direction? Help!

—Crazy in the City

This could have just as easily been signed Screeching in the
Suburbs or Raving in the Rurals. Women all over are feeling the
pain of their hormones gone haywire. I get it, I was there! Let
me tell you my story.

## MY STORY

It crept up on me. It started with little things, little signs I didn't
pay attention to at first. I had always been thin. In fact, growing
up my nickname was "Boney Mahoney," and that was my reality for years, including my five years as Chrissy Snow on *Three's
Company*. I didn't think about being thin because I just always
*was*. In fact, I had been so skinny that in the three years I was
starring in the fabulous Moulin Rouge extravaganza at the Las
Vegas Hilton I wore shorts under my gowns to look fatter! Imagine. Such a problem!

But at around age thirty-five things started to change. I was
exercising constantly while learning new dance numbers and
doing strenuous production numbers for my show. But instead of
slimming down I was getting a little thick around the middle (not
fat, but thick). And my moods changed . . . things that normally
wouldn't bother me would make me flare up angrily, especially
right before my period. This was completely out of character. I
would feel murderous if anyone dared to suggest that I had PMS.

Afterward, as the hormones calmed down, I would feel
ashamed and mortified by the way I had acted and by the things
I had said. But I still didn't "get it." I had no idea I was entering
perimenopause. No one was talking about this major passage,

certainly not our mothers. In fact, it was their big dark secret, the one they suffered through in silence and with good reason; women of my mother's era were routinely sent away to sanitariums if they got too "hysterical." I knew girls whose mothers had been sent away. No one was shocked or outraged, no one questioned it; it was considered sad but "for their own good." Imagine! I, being clueless, just figured that in midlife some women went crazy. In fact, they did in a way, but at that time no one understood what was happening, least of all the medical community.

> What I also didn't know was that a tumor had already begun growing inside my breast. A ticking time bomb! But I wouldn't know about that for another decade. I didn't know then either that perimenopause is our most dangerous time relative to contracting breast cancer. More about both later.

Mood swings, PMS, plus annoying weight gain are part of a *language* that I could not then understand. I didn't know that these symptoms were simply a prelude to other changes I was about to experience. I didn't know the misery that was coming.

### No One Warned Me I Was About to Lose "*Me*"!

My life was good. I was grateful. My TV success had been so unexpected and glorious. I had everything to be happy about. A wonderful husband, a wonderful son, and finally as a family we were working through the barriers of misunderstandings that had been plaguing ours, like so many others at that time who were trying to blend together children who didn't want new parents or a new "family." It was new and uncharted territory.

Blending our family was a lot of work. I have to say there were many nights I would lie in the dark wondering if it was all worth it. I have to say also that, in retrospect, during the time we were blending our family, not only were *my* hormones changing but they were also colliding with my teenage stepdaughter's hormones. She was sixteen and the combination of the two of us going through severe hormonal changes was awful.

Looking back, I feel terrible I had so little understanding of what was happening to both of us at that time. Had I known anything about it I would have been able to help her and help myself at the same time. Ironically every story line we did on *Three's Company* was about a misunderstanding, and at home misunderstandings were our running theme. Not easy.

I had had a rocky start in life, an abusive alcoholic father, exacerbated by nights filled with fear. By contrast, my adult life was wonderful and beyond my wildest expectations. Professionally, I was enjoying tremendous success, and personally, I luxuriated in a love affair with my husband that I had never known was possible. Putting our two families together was the difficult part; feelings were fragile all around, but years of hard work was paying off. We were making it . . . then came perimenopause!

By nature, I'm a happy, upbeat person. I love life and even in the worst of times I tend to look at all situations as a "glass half full." But now it was beginning to become harder and harder to feel happy or upbeat or loving or funny. I was white-knuckling through every day.

I went from doctor to doctor, getting the same explanations, "It's a passage, dear, it will pass!" No, I would say, "It's not passing!"

*"Take this antidepressant, dear, it will make you feel better."*

*"Take this sleeping pill, it will help you sleep."*

*"Take this antianxiety pill and everything will be okay."*

*"Oops. Your blood pressure is going up. Here's some medication. Oops! Your cholesterol is off. Here's another pill."*

I didn't want their drugs! There had to be another way. I didn't know what, but I had to find some answer because I was falling apart!

Are you relating?

It got worse, I found myself "pissed off" most the time. What happened to *me*? Where was "*I*"? Where had "*I*" gone? I found myself crying (a lot), I was unhappy, and now I was getting fat. I had the fun experience of having the *National Enquirer* print candid pictures of me saying, "Her suit looks snug." That's what I needed, feeling like crap every day and now I had the tabloids commenting on every new fat little inch on my once perfect body. I would look at old *Three's Company* reruns and all I could see was how thin I was. Instead of laughing and enjoying the fun of the show, I was fixated by my adorable teeny little waistline.

I felt like the good times in my life were over. I felt miserable. And I took it out on my incredible husband. It's hard to be Mrs. Wonderful when you haven't slept for three years. My eyes looked tired and worn out, with dark circles underneath them from adrenal burnout. At that time I had no idea how important the adrenals were to health and well-being. To compensate, I'd pile on more concealer.

One day I snapped at Alan for something minuscule and stupid and he got quiet, very quiet, then he said, "You know, Suzanne, a marriage can only take so much of this."

Oh my God! Now I was pushing away the best thing in my life: my pal, my lover, my best friend, my business partner, my husband.

I knew I had to get a grip.

I went from doctor to doctor looking for someone, anyone, who knew the answer to this premenopausal nightmare. I was stunned by the ignorance. No one, not one doctor had a clue how to help me that didn't include drugs. I was offered synthetic hormones.

"But these give you cancer!" I said.

"It's all we've got, dear," is what I heard repeatedly. (If one more doctor called me "dear," I was going to get a gun.)

Then I heard about an endocrinologist in Santa Barbara (from my manicurist, bless her) who was giving women something called bioidentical hormones. I did my blood work in advance, and on the day of my appointment I drove up the Pacific Coast Highway at full speed to maybe find relief.

The doctor said to me, "You poor thing."

"What?" I asked, almost in tears.

"You have almost no progesterone. Your ratio is completely off, and your estrogen is way too low," she said. "You must feel terrible."

"I do!" I wailed pathetically.

What I didn't and couldn't know right then was that this was *the moment* when my life was going to turn around.

That was fifteen years ago.

## NOW, IT'S YOUR TURN

So now, *you* are there. You are feeling similar symptoms and they are disrupting your life. That's why you are reading this book, to find an answer and get some help. Let me tell you right now . . .

### It's All Going to Be Okay!

Just know this; the way you've been feeling (and acting) is not your fault. Hormones are in control of us physically and emotionally. PMS? It feels *real*, right? It is. Your chemicals are messed up and *we are our chemicals*!

Now these little chemical messengers are running are all over the place. But just knowing it's not your fault won't make you feel better. I'm sure you feel terrible about your behavior, like I used to feel the next day, when things calmed down. But I'll tell you:

## It's Not You. It's Your Hormones!

What I'm saying right now is very important; what we do when we have these outbursts is damaging. It's not your fault—you have not been educated in body chemistry—but nonetheless, these flare-ups wound and hurt the ones you love. When you find it in your heart (and pride), apologize! Explain to your loved one(s) how out of control you've been feeling. Promise that you are now on a path to wellness and that it's all going to be okay again. I cannot stress the importance and healing of this simple first step.

You must also know this; you are not alone. Men experience declining hormones also, but they are reluctant (and often clueless) to talk about their symptoms. (Most older men—starting in their late forties and early fifties—have no idea that the belly hanging over their belt, their sagging shoulders and loss of muscle tone, high cholesterol, or multiple heart medications have anything to do with hormones.)

We women begin to lose optimal levels of our female hormones (estrogen and progesterone) during perimenopause, which can last for ten to twelve years before menopause, when there is an almost sudden drop in all our hormones. That's why the effect is so, as they say, "in your face." Men have it a little easier, although the outcome reached is similar. On an emotional level, testosterone is what gives men their enthusiasm and confidence. When it drops too low they experience the blues and grumpiness just like we do.

At present the orthodox medical community doesn't accept

that there are safe, effective, natural ways to deal with this challenging passage. They deal with the symptoms of this life transition by prescribing various drugs, what I call the Band-Aid approach. But these solutions promote other negative health changes in women and men, and cause many other conditions to worsen as a result.

This is the book you've been waiting for. I've been there and survived and I am now enjoying superb health and an incredible quality of life; in fact, my experience is joyous.

You too can enjoy perimenopause! Yes, I said enjoy and I mean it.

I will explain what I did, whom I learned from, and what you can expect. It's all good. You are going to be fine; in fact, your life will be better in most cases than ever before. This book will guide you through this difficult and confusing passage.

You are about to get your life back. You are about to be able to enjoy each day and wake up happy and balanced. You are about to realize that this next passage brings with it confidence, joy, and wisdom. You are about to enter the best time of your life. What you have been experiencing—not understanding your feelings, your moods, your body changes, your lack of control—has been devastating.

You want better. You deserve better.

Your answers are here. Say good-bye to the Band-Aid approach of traditional medicine. You are going to have energy, vitality, without drugs. You are going to feel like having sex again (even if right now you don't think you care), your moods are going to stabilize, and your weight will normalize. You are going to be okay, and you are going to be healthy . . . very healthy. Stay with me.

The health issues you face are fixable by restoring hormones the natural way. No matter your age or gender, restoring your hormones to their optimal healthy levels has the same effect as giving water to a dying plant.

Before we go any further, let's take a peek at exactly what's going on inside the female body during our different life transitions.

# CHAPTER 1

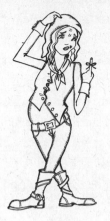

# CHANGE, CHANGE, CHANGE—
# A BASIC LOOK AT OUR BODIES AND
# THEIR TRANSITIONS

Laugh and the world laughs with you. Cry and
you cry with your girlfriends.

—Laurie Kuslansky

Today, looking at my granddaughters as they enter puberty I understand from my own life experience that they can't know that the ease of their little girl lives is now going to start becoming complicated. Chemical changes and life itself become very difficult to understand. This is the life cycle. As we enter womanhood we grow breasts, our moods change, our bodies change, the *known* is now *unknown*, uncharted new territory.

Becoming a woman, especially *before you are a woman*, is a difficult passage at best. There is so much pressure. You may be the first one in your class to get your period, or the last one; both scenarios feel awful. You may be the one with the huge boobs, or the one whose breasts have not grown at all and the boys notice. Again, either way, other kids make fun of you, and you feel mortified.

I was the last in my class to grow breasts and the last to get my period. I was so embarrassed by this that I pretended I had my period when I really didn't just so I wasn't *the* one who was *"out of the group."* I made up stories about my "cramps" like the other girls. There was always some girl in the class who had cramps so bad, real or imagined, that she had to be sent home. I wished so much then that it could be me. (Imagine.)

One day, the other girls found out I was lying when my mother, who did not know how to tell a lie or be dishonest, told the mother of the most popular girl in the class that she didn't know why I was such a late bloomer.

The word was out and they all made fun of me. "How could you?" I wailed to my perplexed mother.

The year before this, the Catholic school I attended started running those scratchy black-and-white films showing sterile pictures of fallopian tubes and talking about "bleeding." *Eeewww!* I didn't want to know anything about it, at the time, which is pretty funny considering my work now. But I digress. So there I was, the only one in my class without her period and wishing/ praying for it!

It all seems silly now, but so overwhelming when you are a fifteen-year-old.

Why did I even want the process to begin? I had the freedom of living without hormonal cycles, and the relatively steady physical and emotional balance of that freedom. Yet I did not know to appreciate it. No one told me about the long, drawn-out process I was about to enter; I did not know of the cycles of woman.

Then it finally came . . . a spot of blood. I was thrilled! "Guess what?" I blurted out to my mother. "I'm bleeding!" She seemed embarrassed, but later that evening without a mention she put a box of Kotex (trade name for humongous sanitary pads) in my room along with this awful-looking strap-thing-y to hold it on to my skinny little body. It felt like I was riding a horse, but I wore it proudly and complained about the discomfort to my girlfriends (for attention) while I prayed for cramps.

My mother was very Victorian, modest and shy, so she never really talked to me about it. In fact, the entire "sex talk" we had happened one day when I was standing on the kitchen stool putting away some dishes for her on a high shelf. She remarked that I had some hair under my arms (about four strands), and then she whispered, "Oh, do you have it *down there* also?"

*Down there.* That was it; the closest we ever got to talking about my changing body, my transition, my new life. A product of her time, my mother's shame of her own body became my shame, so I kept all things girly and personal to myself.

I entered womanhood having no idea of what it meant.

## A PEEK UNDER THE HOOD

The female body is miraculous and complex, capable of bringing new life into the world by way of our reproductive organs. But what exactly goes on "down there" and in there? It's important to understand how our bodies work: our exquisite female reproductive system consists of internal and external parts.

The external parts include the labia majora and the labia minora, also called lips, that surround the vagina and urethra and protect the internal organs from infectious organisms. The internal parts include the vagina, which claims both the functions of enabling sperm to enter the woman's body and being a birth canal. The uterus is the organ that carries a growing fetus, and the cervix is the lower part of the uterus that joins the uterus and the vagina. The ovaries, which rest to either side, produce eggs, and the fallopian tubes allow eggs to travel into the uterus.

Our bodies are magnificent. Each month we experience apoptosis, a fancy name for the necessary death of cells. We can understand this better by an explanation of our monthly period and what happens in the uterus. Each month we shed the lining of the endometrium (cell death) and it is cleared from our bodies through the process called menstruation. This monthly bleed is a necessary form of cell death to make way for new cells and to remove cells whose DNA has been damaged to the point at which cancerous change is liable to occur. It's a brilliant process, always clearing our bodies monthly to keep us healthy; it is only interrupted if we become pregnant, and in that case the endometrium lining holds the nourishment for the developing fetus.

If an egg released from the ovaries is fertilized by sperm, and pregnancy occurs, it will travel through the fallopian tube and implant itself in the uterus. During pregnancy, the egg, or embryo, grows into a fetus inside the uterus, which expands in size to accommodate the developing baby. A woman carries the baby in her uterus, or womb, until the baby is ready to be born.

When a woman's body expels all the eggs produced by the ovaries during the course of her lifetime, menopause begins and the ability to reproduce ends. Menopause should really be called "egglessness." It's a friendlier term. Before we get to eggless, however, our hormones begin to decline subtly, in what we call perimenopause. Meaning you can still reproduce but it will become more difficult to conceive, difficult to carry to full term, and the eggs left are often not as strong and healthy. Sometimes, but not always, this leaves babies born to moms at risk for birth defects and health conditions.

As fully reproductive women we make enough estrogen each month so that it reaches its peak on the twelfth day, stops the growth of cells, and makes progesterone receptors. Without an estrogen peak, your brain can't send the signal to release any of the eggs you have left. With no estrogen peak there's no feedback information to shut off follicle-stimulating hormone, so FSH pours constantly, overstimulating your ovaries and ripening all at once most of the eggs you have left. The loss of this rhythm in perimenopause actually triggers the destruction of the rest of your eggs through the action of excessive FSH, using up the remainder of your eggs. At about this time, you begin to feel the heat of hot flashes. That's how the system effectively shuts itself down for good. This process can take a decade— a *long* uncomfortable decade!

This is all background to explain why the healthiest woman is a reproductive woman, and once hormones begin to decline, new science has proved that replacing the missing hormones restores a woman to her healthiest prime even though she is no longer capable of making a baby.

What I did know was that now I felt different. I was getting used to the ups and downs of the surges of sex hormones and menstrual cycles, as well as the (very welcome) growth of pubic hair, breasts, and sex feelings. Now I felt that I was like all the other girls.

But then my breasts kept growing. (Wow, be careful what you wish for!) I started out at fifteen wearing a scant 32A cup (padded), hardly filling it, and by the summer of my sixteenth year I was an overflowing 34C that could hardly be contained. My breasts grew so big and so fast on my skinny little body that they were a little embarrassing, but I liked the attention I was getting from having them, including attention from my lecherous drama teacher who would say highly inappropriate things to me when no one was around. I got the part of Adelaide in *Guys and Dolls* partly due to my talent, partly due to my shapely, curvy body, and partly because that lecherous one wanted me around. My father didn't like the new me at all. My body seemed to make him angry, and he would say things like, "For chrissakes, put some clothes on."

## BYE-BYE PUBERTY

Transitioning into womanhood, like all transitions, is an agitating and confusing experience. It's a long, bumpy, uncomfortable road; but then you adjust to the excitement, privileges, and challenges of being an adult. This is also a time when your hormones reach their maximum. By the time you are in your twenties and thirties, you enter a period of remarkable high energy, clear thinking, and all the drama of being an adult and building your adult life. You don't quite know who you are yet in most cases, but you sure are having fun. Your body is the best looking it will ever be; your breasts are high and perky, and your sex drive is off the charts. You are oozing estrogen. For most people this is a time of perfect hormonal balance. Diet affects your hormones at this time like any time, but your youth withstands the assault of binge drinking, hangovers, fast food, quarts of ice cream, and sugary desserts. Somehow you sleep it off, bang down giant cups of coffee, and sail through work until the end of the next week, when you do it to yourself all over again.

## HELLO, MIDLIFE . . .

Sometime between your midthirties and midforties another series of physical changes begins to takes place. Transitions! In general, this is a time of strength and vibrancy, but now you are more affected by outside factors and lifestyle choices. And as I just said, things are shifting again. Your periods may become a little erratic, your breasts may get painfully lumpy, and sometimes your periods get lighter or heavier than usual, or you are bleeding between them. You or your friends may be struggling with: infertility, difficulty conceiving or carrying a pregnancy to term, endometriosis, uterine fibroids, sudden weight gain, foggy thinking, memory loss, migraine headaches, cold hands and/or feet, and premenstrual syndrome, even when you've never had it before.

You are a little moodier than you used to be and you tire more easily. The kids can get on your nerves in ways they never had before. By the end of the day you can't wait for that 5:00 cocktail to cool out and relax. You don't recover from a long trip or a night out as easily, either, and staying home becomes more alluring than constantly running to the next event. You need more sleep, but the sleep you are getting isn't as sound as it once was. Your muscles strain more easily when you are working out, and when you get out of bed in the morning, you might grunt a little from the stiffness. The fast food you enjoyed in your twenties now gives you heartburn, and drink one too many glasses of wine and you will have a whopper of a headache.

But the big one . . . you don't feel like having sex the way you used to. Is it you? Is it him? You don't know, but it's depressing and it takes its toll around the house.

Your husband is working as hard as he can to give you the lifestyle you both want. You likely are working two jobs: in your career and at home. You feel "put upon" because he is always gone and you have to do everything. He doesn't seem to realize all you do and that you are working from morning till late at night being the perfect mom, wife, housekeeper, career woman, and preparing for everyone for the next day while *he's* already asleep under the covers with the TV blaring. You can't help it when you get annoyed that he didn't stay up for you, even though he has an early morning appointment. Could this be PMS? No, you say to yourself. This is real. It's him. You start to have dark thoughts about breaking out, getting away. But these are just fantasies . . . aren't they? Your PMS used to be mild, but now it can carry with it a surge of fury. Plus, you've gained a little weight and you can't seem to exercise enough to get it off. That too is annoying. You ask him if what you're wearing makes you look fat, and if he says yes, it's an evening wrecker.

What is happening? You are now at midtransition. Fun, huh?

## HORMONE HELL

Just like with puberty, now your hormones seem to be all over the place again. Just when you had gotten used to feeling great all the time, it's like something has stripped it away. Your hormones are fluctuating up and down, like they have a mind of their own, but the overall direction of them is down, just as your reproductive years are winding down.

In puberty your hormones fluctuate, which is why you cry, yell at your mother, get depressed and feel suicidal if your boyfriend breaks up with you. Plus you hate your body and you feel fat, and your parents are mean and no one understands you.

Then you transition through that passage into your reproductive years and suddenly your cycles are regular. You feel happy and serene, and proud of your abilities to reproduce. And aren't you something that you have given birth to these incredible children? They are perfect and so is your life. Your husband brings you flowers, and you have great standing-up sex in the shower with the door locked, while the kids are still safely sleeping in their rooms. Life is good. Life is smooth sailing and delicious.

Then along comes perimenopause and the fluctuations start

again, almost like you are back in puberty. You cry for no reason, no one understands you, you are overworked and underappreciated, your body is betraying you, and did I mention, no one in the house understands you?

You are on your way to menopause, something you don't even want to think about because you haven't even figured out perimenopause. How could you be experiencing it anyway, as you feel you are way too young for this. Aren't you?

Eventually you will transition into menopause where your hormones are just low and steady, maybe leaving you feeling flat and lifeless.

This is being a woman! It ain't for sissies, and it's why we're so strong. Don't worry. You are going to be just fine once you learn how to take care of yourself through this major transition.

It's very exciting to know that today we have emerging science and cutting-edge doctors who have stepped out of the dark and into a new light, declaring the status quo to be obsolete. There is a solution, a healthy and pleasant way to make all the transitions of your life something you will look forward to experiencing. This new approach is backed up by science and clinical studies and is great news for young women; you do not have to go through all the ups and downs associated with perimenopause and eventually menopause. These life transitions can be made enjoyable, if you know what to do.

The new approach is about knowledge and the power that accompanies knowledge. Clearly, lifestyle shifts relative to diet, sleep, and exercise are crucial, but the advancements made in natural hormone replacement are the new game changer. This book is meant to inform you about what is happening in your body and clearly show you the safety and efficacy of natural hormone replacement, giving you many options to take away any fears you may have surrounding their use.

This book offers hope. You can sail through your transitions and enjoy the quality of life I am enjoying. You can make each new passage upbeat, comfortable, and sexy, if you take advantage of this new thinking.

Now that we know how it all works, that we females are complex and fabulous, let's more closely investigate why you are feeling the way you've been feeling and look at the symptoms that are part of the process we call perimenopause.

# CHAPTER 2

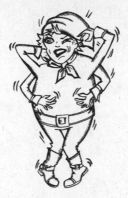

# IT STARTED WITH AN ITCH— COMMON SYMPTOMS OF PERIMENOPAUSE

Thirty-five is when you finally get your head together and your body starts falling apart.
—Caryn Leschen

It started with an itch! A maddening, "drive you crazy" kind of itch; I'd try not to scratch, but eventually I always gave in. My legs were a mess. I couldn't figure it out. What was causing this? I figured I had some kind of allergy that even anti-itch creams couldn't seem to help. My doctors didn't connect it to hormonal decline.

Then, as I explained earlier, I lost control of my moods. When Alan confronted me, I was mortified and terrified. Had I been acting that badly? Was I "flying off the handle" that often? Was I taking out my bad mood on him *that frequently*? I'm going to shamefully admit to all the above. I also have to say this moment with Alan got my attention. I was putting our solid, loving, unbelievably wonderful love affair in jeopardy. I certainly did not want to do that.

In my first books on hormones, I labeled the common symptoms that erupt during menopause as the Seven Dwarves:

1. Itchy
2. Bitchy
3. Sleepy
4. Sweaty
5. Bloated
6. Forgetful
7. All Dried Up

Well, those dwarves might be smaller during perimenopause, but they are still as mighty!

Dwarf #2, Bitchy, had taken up full-time residence in our house. My sunny disposition was gone. It's hard to have a big smile on your face when you can only sleep three hours nightly, and you are sweating and tossing and turning, first hot then cold. Not to mention that constant "noise" in your head that won't shut up, as well as a total loss of sexual desire (remember Dwarf #7, All Dried Up?). Yes, I did feel crazy, because I didn't want to act this way. I wanted things to be as they had been before. But I didn't feel in control and to add insult to injury, Dwarf #5, Bloated, was with me all the time!

I went from doctor to doctor and I was offered every drug available: antidepressants, antianxiety meds, sleeping pills, blood pressure pills, cholesterol medications. One old doctor even patted me on the back and said, "The drug companies know best, dear."

Oh my. That's when I knew I was on my own. I did not want

to go down that path of the women I watched before me who were on the "menopause cocktail" of drugs that conveniently shut them up. Prozac, after all, may make you feel better. But you don't have a Prozac deficiency, you have a hormone deficiency!

Foggy brains and brittle bones have been the experience women have observed in their other friends so they feel it is normal; miserable, but normal. Women deal with their misery by going to lunch and commiserating with each other. They drink too much wine and get happy laughing about their symptoms. Oops! Senior moment! Hello, Dwarf #6 (Forgetful). Wine makes you temporarily feel good; and women are starving to feel good and to be understood, if only for a couple of hours at lunch. But too much wine does backfire as you'll read a little later, resulting in more weight gain and, because it has yeast, more bloating and discomfort.

## YOU'RE NOT CRAZY, THIS IS NORMAL

Hormonal loss can indeed make you feel like you are going crazy. You don't know who you are anymore, and you can't rely on feeling good each day. Perimenopause is the transitional stage from normal menstrual periods to no periods at all. It may start in your thirties or forties and it will continue until you reach the final stage, menopause, probably sometime in your fifties. You are transitioning. This process and the cluster of symptoms that often come with it can start ten years before actual full-blown menopause.

Perimenopause is a natural phase of life, and in many cases it is a difficult transition. When you don't understand what's happening and don't know how to manage it, or *if* you can manage it, then your health and your sanity can be challenged.

Long before your final period, your hormones start to become amazingly unpredictable. That final period comes at the end of the process, not the beginning. This is why it is so confusing to young women. How could they be in perimenopause when they still have their monthly bleed?

The discomfort and symptoms you are feeling are all a result of declining and shifting hormones in your body, and these little messengers cause an array of symptoms we'll fully explore in this chapter. Before we do, let's first talk a little about this term you hear so often but that you may not yet fully understand: hormones.

## WHAT ARE HORMONES?

What are they? Does everyone have them? Why do we need them? These are the questions I am asked over and over. It is truly amazing to me that substances so crucial to the efficient working of the human body, the substances responsible for your quality of life, are so misunderstood and so little is known about them.

This is your primer on the hormonal system; it's very important you know what they are, what they do, and why you need them. I've tried to keep this information simple. Having this knowledge will empower you to understand your body and transform your experience of this transition.

Every human body on the planet has hormones. Hormones build bones, maintain muscle tone, and protect your joints. They regulate your heartbeat and breathing. Hormones fight stress, calm anxiety, relieve depression, and allow you to *feel*. Hormones govern your sex drive and fertility. They stimulate your brain and immune system, and relieve pain. They govern the menstrual cycle and they allow for pregnancy.

When they are in balance, you feel perfect. When they are out of balance, your life quality diminishes substantially.

The hormones estrogen, progesterone, and testosterone make us men and women. Every woman and man has different hormonal requirements. That's why there is no "one pill fits all" solution. Your hormonal requirements are unique. What you need is different from what I need.

This is what hormones "do"; now you might be wondering what they are made of—what they are exactly? A hormone is a chemical substance produced in your body by your glands. They are a complex combination of chemical keys that turn important metabolic locks in our cells, tissues, and organs. All the approximately sixty to ninety trillion cells in our bodies are influenced to some degree by these amazing hormonal keys.

The turning on of these "locks" stimulates activity within the cells of our brain, intestines, muscles, genital organs, and skin. As such, hormones determine the rate at which our cells burn up nutrients and other food substances, release energy, and determine whether our cells should produce milk, hair, secretions, enzymes, or some other metabolic (life) product. Hormones affect virtually every function in your body. They affect your mood, how you cope, your sexuality, your sex drive. We all have hormones and without them we would simply die. From the moment we are born, our hormones play a major role in how we grow, age, and function.

All our hormones depend on one another. They have an interactive "language" and work as a team to maintain our health. If one is missing or insufficient, this will affect the other hormones. Imbalanced hormones are a setup for disease and health problems. Notice that things go "wrong" at the end of our reproductive years. Remember (and my longtime readers know this): biologically we are here to make babies (perpetuate the species) and then get out of the way when we are no longer able to do so.

We get sick when one or more members of the hormone team are not working at the same capacity as the other hormones. So when your doctor says "Your thyroid is a little low," it's a big deal. It's a sign of imbalance. But why do our hormones decline or get off balance in the first place?

Hormones decline when the endocrine glands cannot maintain the same production of hormones you were making in your younger years. The loss of hormones can begin as early as the midtwenties (Imagine!), but generally at around age thirty-five is when you start to feel their loss. Yes, it happens that young. Declining hormone levels accelerate the aging process. The toxins in the environment are also big factors in this decline and the acceleration of aging, but they are rarely connected to hormone loss by mainstream medicine.

## SLUGGISH, AGING, AND SAD

With hormonal decline come withdrawal symptoms. The symptoms vary from woman to woman, but the symptoms are all part of the process—a very uncomfortable one at that. It's similar to what you experienced in puberty when your hormone levels were rising. Except now, in perimenopause, the situation is reversing and the people around you are not so understanding; you're supposed to behave like a "grown-up" after all. On the way down you are going to experience the same emotional and physical havoc you experienced when your hormones first started building up. It's no fun.

It's like your body suddenly betrays you. It does. In some cases, hormone loss can progress to major disability, deformity, pain, disease, and depression. Yet most conventional doctors never connect these dots. What is even more unimaginable to me, though, are the women who choose to do nothing about it and allow their health to deteriorate.

As we decline in hormone production we slow down. Our bodies get sluggish in every way, which sets you up for some form of what modern medicine calls "age-related" illness—even if you are still young!

Sadly, many of us accept this so-called aging as normal or inevitable. Even sadder is the lack of understanding on the part of many doctors, so that women have to endure this passage: suffering with fluctuating moods, serial anxiety, an inability to cope, and destructive behaviors that can ruin marriages in many instances. Many accept the debilitating symptoms of hormone decline as an unavoidable way of life. This is often compounded by misinformed, but well-meaning doctors telling us that this is all normal "for our age."

Says who?

## IS THIS YOUR LIFE?—
## IT DOESN'T HAVE TO BE

We'll come back a little later to hormones and what each major and minor hormone does in the body. For now, let's talk about some of the discomforts you may be experiencing, and why they shouldn't be taken lightly.

Up first: PMS.

### PMS (aka, Being Bitchy)

I had it bad.

Real bad.

Jekyll and Hyde bad!

Like I said before, when you don't sleep for months and years on end, you are tired . . . and cranky! But it's a different kind of cranky because there is no logic to it. You fly off the handle and then the next day you know in your heart that you overreacted, but it's so embarrassing to once again apologize for being a bitch. This is when you feel like you are going crazy, a very disconcerting feeling.

About a third of all women suffer with PMS to varying degrees. PMS usually occurs two weeks before your period and stops when bleeding begins. Its symptoms get worse as you age. In our twenties and thirties, our estradiol levels gracefully rise during the course of a month from a low of about 30 pg/dL (picograms per deciliter) right before a period to a high of about 400 pg/dL right before ovulation. The effects of this dramatic drop in a woman's estradiol levels are what we usually call PMS. In perimenopause, however, these levels may vary and unpredictably spike into the thousands with totally unnerving side effects, the most common of which are breast tenderness, breast lumps, headaches, cramps, fatigue, bloating, water retention, weight gain, crankiness (or worse), forgetfulness, insomnia, anger, depression, and mood swings. Nice, huh?

When menopause arrives, levels may crash to as low as 10 or 15 pg/dL. That was where I found myself on the day I finally found a doctor (after searching for three long years) who understood bioidentical hormone replacement. It was humiliating to sit in her office weeping as she patted my head and told me it was all going to be okay.

Adrenal burnout caused by stress can exacerbate PMS. (And stress is always involved with PMS.) Thyroid abnormalities also play a role in PMS symptoms. Both affect pituitary output; the pituitary is the hormone contractor telling all the other hormones what to do. We'll get into the roles of the major and minor hormones more in coming chapters. Essentially, what you are talking about is that for many women, perimenopause is like an internal train wreck.

Frankly, PMS is part of the language I refer to so often in my books. It's your body telling you "all is not well." Unpleasant as it may be, think of PMS as an internal friend telling you to get to the bottom of your issues to head off serious problems down the road.

## Weight Gain

One of the most common complaints of perimenopause is unexplained weight gain. You start getting "thick," especially around the middle. Your belly bloats and you retain water, even when you never did before. You may eat less and exercise more yet you still can't lose the weight; instead, often you gain weight.

Low thyroid, a major hormone (which we will explore in depth in chapter 4) is usually the culprit. When it's too low, you don't metabolize food effectively and the calories you consume turn into fat instead of energy; this is why exercising and dieting helps a little, but you just can't achieve the weight loss you desire.

Low thyroid weight tends to be distributed evenly on your body. When low pituitary function is at the root of your low thyroid function it's generally confined to the area from your abdomen to just above your knees. (If you ever hit your head as a kid or in an accident as an adult, it would be good to have your pituitary levels checked. These injuries—especially multiple concussions—can jostle your pituitary and make for hormonal issues later in life, especially thyroid issues; see Ives.) Ensuring that you take in sufficient essential fatty acids (omega-3 fish oil) will help with weight loss.

## Foggy Thinking and Forgetfulness

One of the most common complaints of hormonal decline (and fears) is "foggy thinking." Right next to it is its sister, forgetfulness. I remember when it began happening to me. I couldn't think. Sometimes I couldn't remember the end of the sentence I was about to speak. I would go blank while being interviewed on TV, so I developed a clever way of "changing the subject" so as not to be embarrassed.

This phenomenon is due to estrogen loss to the brain, which takes the first "hit" in declining hormones. I know you feel you are too young to be thinking about your brain, but look down the road; don't you think all those women ahead of you with dementia or worse now wish they had taken brain health seriously?

This brain fog is a result of a complex series of events that happens to women.

First, it's about estrogen depletion. The brain needs estrogen to function properly. When a woman is deficient in estrogen, she develops senior moments or brain farts—whatever description you can handle to take the edge off your embarrassment with your friends and make for a big laugh. You may be laughing off your embarrassment on the outside, but on the inside there is nothing funny about it.

When it happened to me, I secretly harbored a fear that this was the first stage of Alzheimer's, the most frightening of all diseases to me. Estrogen depletion also causes headaches and migraines. What is least known, though, is the connection that brain fog and depression have to the GI tract. Seventy percent of your immune system is made in the GI tract (*see* Vighi). When the gut becomes inflamed due to overuse of antibiotics, food allergies or food intolerances, toxins, fluoride, chlorine, benzene, PCBs, poor food choices, and over-the-counter or prescription drugs, the immune system downgrades. It then limits or ceases serotonin production.

Serotonin is a hormone and is the relaxing brain chemical made primarily in the intestines but also profoundly affects the brain, where it impacts brain cells by various mechanisms (*see* Hadhazy). Serotonin activity is essential for enjoying a relaxed and happy brain. This is the feel-good hormone that speaks directly to the pleasure center of your brain. Altered serotonin metabolism may be associated with many conditions, including: gut disturbances, yeast infections, bodily aches, foggy thinking, and depression.

Our female hormones are very potent modulators of the brain chemicals dopamine, serotonin, and GABA. According to Dr. Rick Sponaugle, an environmental medical specialist, when a woman's hormones are out of balance, so is the electrical activity of her brain. PMS symptoms are really an indicator of serotonin deficiency, and because her levels are deficient or low, she will experience depression, anxiety, insomnia, and often brain fog.

Most women at this point need something to take the "pain" of anxiety, worry, and bodily aches away. So they go to alcohol or over-the-counter or prescription drugs like Prozac, Oxycontin, or Xanax.

We all know women who can't remember what happened yesterday, who can't hold a thought. They are functioning but slightly "out of it." It's important if you are experiencing any memory lapses to take it seriously. It likely means your hormone levels are starting to decline. Before you start having trouble with your GI tract, your joints, your brain, get some help.

## Hot Flashes

Hot flashes are different from the kind of sweating experienced in hot weather, which helps to cool us down and make us more comfortable. Hot flashes induced by low estrogen cause a cycle of hot skin, sweating, evaporation, and then a clammy chill. They are extremely uncomfortable and, worse, unpredictable. You never know when to expect one. They can occur as many as ten to fifteen times in succession; sometimes this happens at night, sometimes in the middle of the day. That's the unpredictable part.

## Painful, Swollen Breasts

I was plagued by this one. I couldn't wait to take my bra off at the end of the day. When my breasts were set free, they felt like they were these two heavy pendulums that ached with pain. They kept getting bigger and bigger, like the breasts that were going to take over Los Angeles! Out of their harness, I walked around holding them to protect me from the pain. They were lumpy and swollen all the time. (How I wish I knew then that they were simply begging for progesterone and then they would have calmed down.)

At least fifty percent of women suffer from lumpy, swollen, painful breasts, called *fibrocystic breast disease,* at one time or another, and it's one of the most common reasons a woman goes to a doctor. Painful, swollen breasts are indicators of several conditions and thus can be confusing to a woman and her doctor:

- At one time it was thought that fibrocystic breasts predisposed women to cancer, but that turned out to be misleading; in fact, fibrocystic breasts make evaluation of new lumps or abnormal changes more difficult.
- Premenstrual swollen breasts are painful but harmless.
- Constantly lumpy and painful breasts can indicate chronic estrogen dominance, which some alternative health care practitioners claim may increase the risk for breast cancer. These lumps are tender and the pain lasts throughout the month, although at times the pain is worse than at others.
- Cysts are benign or noncancerous and are usually "rubbery" to feel but are often painful.
- Cancerous lumps are usually hard, fixed in location, and typically not painful.

It takes a qualified doctor who acts as a detective to decipher which of these conditions is yours and treat you accordingly.

Consuming excessive caffeine aggravates painful breasts, so it's worth reducing caffeine to see if the pain and swelling subsides.

Painful swollen breasts are part of the "language" of this transition and any of the above scenarios needs checking. I walked around for years with painful lumpy breasts. I never knew what my breasts were trying to tell me until it was too late.

## Yeast Infections

Yeast . . . the new enemy. There's hardly a woman around who hasn't had a yeast infection. It plays havoc in your vagina. Yeast is an overgrowth of *Candida albicans* in the vagina. Yeast overgrowth is very uncomfortable: it causes vaginal itching, burning, redness, soreness, white cottage-cheese-like vaginal discharge, and painful intercourse. What fun is hot sex when your vagina is on fire like this? It gives a whole new meaning to being "hot"!

With overuse of antibiotics, many women upon reaching perimenopause find themselves with recurring yeast infections. Western medicine generally does not prescribe probiotics to accompany antibiotic intake but think about this:

ANTIbiotic takes away.
PRObiotic puts back.

It just makes sense that if an antibiotic is going to take away the balanced flora, a balance so vital to life, digestion, and good health, then taking a probiotic is a no-brainer.

Antibiotics kill the beneficial and harmful bacteria and create pH imbalances that occur in the vagina. Common causes that favor yeast include increased pH, increased heat and moisture, allergic reactions, elevated sugar levels, hormonal imbalances, and reductions in the populations of beneficial bacteria that are normally present. Sex lubricants have also been linked to yeast infections, including the lubricants with the spermicide non-oxynol-9.

Here's where perimenopause comes into play. Ironically, estrogen deficiencies cause carbohydrate (sugar) craving, which is the exact opposite of what your body needs when you have too much yeast. It is part of the merry-go-round: the weight gain, the sugar, chocolate cravings, combing the cupboards at night looking for sweets or toast with butter and lots of sugary jam. These cravings are physical, so it's difficult to resist. Your brain needs a dopamine hit.

Candida can flare up as a result of stress, or drinking too much wine (especially white wine with its high sugar and the yeast inherent in the wine itself). Perimenopausal women often drink a lot of white wine (so do the menopausal ones) because they don't feel good, and a glass of wine in the evening with girlfriends is pleasurable and enjoyable. It takes away the edge, when they are feeling like they are just "holding on." They are white-knuckling each day, and they'd like to let go and blow off steam, but that wouldn't bode well with others, so instead they hold it inside. Stressful!

No wonder a glass of wine soothes the feeling. And while you are out with the girls, why not have a plate of pasta to go with the white wine (white flour = sugar)? What the heck, why not grab a dessert, too? Now the yeast has a perfect meal. It loves sugar. It thrives on sugar. As a result, your vagina is on fire. A night of yeast and sugar, combined with imbalanced hormones (either too much estrogen or too little progesterone, or the reverse) and you've got a little yeast factory growing in your vagina. Then your husband wants sex! I don't think so. You tell him it's out of commission and the merry-go-round goes round and round.

## Breakthrough Bleeding

When hormones begin to decline, many changes take place and breakthrough bleeding is a common (albeit unpleasant) and sometimes frightening occurrence.

Many women report inconsistency with their monthly periods during perimenopause. Sometimes periods are very light; sometimes very heavy. Sometimes they are at their normal "twenty-eight days" for a cycle. Sometimes it's shorter or much, much longer. Trying to find the new "normal" can be tricky.

The majority of irregular periods and irregular bleeding is a sign that you are lacking hormonal balance. For older women, it may be an indicator that you are not achieving an estrogen peak. When I write "older" here, I am referring to women usually in full transition to menopause who aren't making enough of either estrogen or progesterone.

If this is happening to you, go to a qualified doctor and ask to have your hormone levels checked to see if they are high enough and in the right ratios. Don't go to the doctor clueless. You know what is not feeling right and your doctor will appreciate that you are involved with the workings of your body and your desire to get it right.

## Loss of Sex Drive

Did you know that having frequent sex can increase your life expectancy? Being sexually active has many benefits, including stress relief. It is said that frequent orgasms (about a hundred a year) can increase life expectancy by three to eight years. It's a simple equation. If you want to live longer, have more sex! It's that vital to life, and to your emotional well-being.

But what if you just can't *feel* sex anymore? I hear this from

younger women almost daily; they want to feel—they want to
*want* sex—but they just can't and don't.

Don't worry; it's not you. It's not that you are bored with your
partner; it's a physical phenomenon. You have declining or missing sex hormones: estrogen, progesterone, and testosterone.
Without these vital hormones the "feeling" isn't there. (We'll discuss these "minor" hormones in a chapter all their own.)

A healthy person is a sexual person. Perhaps there is no one
in your life you care to share such intimacies with at present, but
that doesn't mean your body should feel dead sexually.

Another factor in diminishing sex drive is stress. Stress is the
biggest romance killer that exists. Stress blunts hormone production. (Hear that, superwomen?) If you combine stress and imbalanced hormones, a good-night kiss could be a chore.

Both women and men will lose their sex hormones in the
aging process, and the negative effects are more prevalent today
than at any other time in the history of humankind. The reasons
are we are living longer and we are living more stressful lives.

Don't worry, there is a solution. Keep reading.

## Headaches

Another symptom of hormonal imbalance is headache. Luckily
this was not one of my symptoms. Headaches, sadly, are part of
the perimenopausal and menopausal experience for so many
women. Women suffer migraines, a particularly debilitating
type of headache, about three times more frequently than men,
affecting up to 60 percent of all women at some point in their
lives. They occur before, during, or immediately after a period,
or during ovulation. They range from mild to "migraine fierce."
Why do these debilitating headaches occur more frequently during perimenopause?

The brain requires estrogen to operate optimally. Low, imbalanced, or fluctuating estrogen levels can trigger migraines; menstrual migraines are primarily caused by estrogen, and when the levels of estrogen and progesterone change, women are more vulnerable to migraine headaches. Too much or too little estrogen causes blood vessels to dilate. If your progesterone is too low to balance your estrogen, leaving you estrogen dominant, the swelling blood vessel dilation caused by unchallenged estrogen can be a catalyst.

Insufficient magnesium levels make arteries more susceptible to spasm and are another common cause of other types of headaches. One possible reason for this deficiency in magnesium is a chronic imbalance of estrogen to progesterone. This imbalance is not only uncomfortable, but a dangerous setup for cancer. Low thyroid can cause headaches, too, as can low adrenal function.

## DID YOU RECOGNIZE YOURSELF ABOVE?

If you are experiencing some or all of these symptoms, you most assuredly are "there." You have entered perimenopause and now it's time to restore your body to its optimal healthy prime. Your life and body will all come back to balance and in many cases be better than ever before. You are going to learn, like me, what to do to really enjoy perimenopause and all the transitions to come.

The fix includes lifestyle, diet, and hormone replacement. You have to understand each of the hormones underlying these symptoms, how they function, and why your body needs them replaced to restore your life and body to balance. So that's what we'll focus on in the next two chapters.

Perimenopause is an exciting time in a woman's life if you choose to look at it optimistically. You have no choice in the matter, as each passing year brings its transitions and changes, whether you like it or not. It's better to go with the flow. Your wisdom is starting to emerge. You've lived long enough to start having some perspective. When you are balanced, these factors allow you to react calmly and with measure to the things in life that up till now would put you over the top. With hormonal balance comes calm, and then contentment. Doesn't that sound worth having? It's within your grasp. Keep reading.

Let's get started. Next up: the minor hormones.

# CHAPTER 3

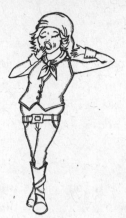

# THE MINOR HORMONES—
# OR WHY YOU'RE FEELING SO CRAPPY

I'm not going to vacuum till Sears makes one
you can ride on.

—Roseanne Barr

If you are in perimenopause, then declines in the hormones—estrogen, progesterone, testosterone, and DHEA (called "minor" hormones by mainstream medicine) and the secondary hormones oxytocin and pregnenolone—are likely prompting your suffering. Withdrawal symptoms are probably why you picked up this book. Because you just don't feel right!

Why these hormones are called minor I'll never know. When these are off, declining, or missing, there is nothing minor about the way you feel. The minor hormones allow for your quality of life. When your minors go into a decline, your majors (thyroid,

insulin, adrenal, cortisol) rise. (More about the majors to come.)
That's why you are feeling inner chaos. Things aren't in balance.

So many women before you have chosen to live a life with
no quality. They have endured sleepless nights, sweaty bodies,
lack of sexual desire, bloated stomachs, itches, and absentmind-
edness (senior moments) because they thought they had no good
choices available. Or they decided to "tough it out." Toughing it
out is a waste of time and potentially dangerous to your health.
It is not noble to suffer this way, regardless of how hard you are
trying to make it so.

Without hormones your body is in a vulnerable state. Remember, nature wants to get rid of you now that you can't perpetuate
the species. Without hormones it's a gradual deterioration, allowing your body parts to slowly wear out. Don't let this happen.

I realize you are not thinking about your old age, but now *is*
the time to start "tricking" your body into thinking you are still
reproductive. That's what this is about. What? you say. Tricking
my body? Yes. If technology is tricking our bodies into living longer with MRIs, CAT scans, sophisticated blood tests, antibiotics,
even sewage disposal systems, then why wouldn't you trick your
body into having "quality of life" in these extra years?

And how thrilling! With balanced hormones you can enjoy
your life, with a rockin' libido and a good figure. There's no free
lunch, though. A good diet and lifestyle habits are part of the program. You can also expect great health, a good working brain (no
senior moments), and the wisdom and perspective that comes
from life experience.

Who doesn't want that? And you won't feel the way you've
been feeling. Sound good?

Understanding the roles that each of the minor hormones
plays in determining your mood, health, and general well-being
is key to learning how to fix them. Then you can sail through

perimenopause. Let's start with progesterone, the "feel good" hormone that usually drops first in perimenopausal women.

## Progesterone

Progesterone is one of the two main hormones produced in the ovaries. The other, of course, is estrogen. Along with estrogen, progesterone prepares the lining of the uterus for pregnancy.

Progesterone levels are low during the first phase of your menstrual cycle (follicular cycle). Levels increase sharply for a maximum of ten days following ovulation, which occurs around day 14. Levels decline rapidly about four days prior to menstruation. This is the rhythm of your body. Your chemicals move up and down throughout the month. As women we can all feel this; different days make us feel different.

As stated above, progesterone is primarily produced in the second half of a woman's menstrual cycle. Reproductively speaking, it is the hormone responsible for the survival of the fetus in pregnancy. Progesterone is also produced in small amounts in the adrenal glands in both sexes (men also produce some progesterone in the testes), where it acts as a precursor for other steroid hormones. (All hormones are considered steroid hormones: testosterone, progesterone, estrogen, DHEA, pregnenolone, aldosterone, and more. The term steroid describes both hormones produced by the body and artificially produced medications that duplicate the action for the naturally occurring steroids.)

The benefits and roles of progesterone are many, including:

- Is a precursor to other sex hormones
- Is essential for pregnancy and the survival of the fetus
- Supports sex drive
- Prevents PMS

- Protects against fibrocystic breasts
- Restores proper cell oxygen levels
- Acts as a natural diuretic
- Protects against endometrial cancer
- Normalizes zinc and copper levels
- Helps counteract the role of estrogen in breast cancer
- Acts as a natural antidepressant
- Normalizes blood clotting
- Facilitates thyroid function
- Helps regulate blood sugar levels
- Stimulates cells for bone building
- Improves energy, stamina, and endurance

In other words, progesterone does a lot. Without it we are left with unopposed estrogen, which will leave you pretty defenseless against disease, including cancer. When progesterone declines severely, we are at risk for having our bodies in an unhealthy hormonal state of imbalance, where excess estrogen, or estrogen dominance, is the norm. Perimenopausal women tend to lose progesterone and deficiency of this hormone leaves us with very "in your face" symptoms, including:

- Painful, tender, swollen breasts
- Anxiety and stress
- Infertility
- Abdominal cramps
- Aggression
- Extremely heavy periods
- PMS
- Night sweats
- Early miscarriage
- Weepiness
- Trouble sleeping

- Headaches associated with your period
- Low bone density
- Weight gain
- Swollen extremities
- Excessive water retention

When I was in my late thirties and early forties, I had pretty much every symptom mentioned. I even remember going to doctor after doctor complaining about my painful swollen breasts and no one understood what to do about it or what it meant.

Perimenopause is problematic biologically because as far as the brain is concerned it thinks the woman is hormonally in the first trimester of pregnancy because of her hormone ranges. The specific hormonal environment of early pregnancy is one of high insulin, coupled with low estrogen and thyroid functioning. These levels are also mimicked in perimenopause. This is why weight gain is so prevalent. The body is confused. It thinks it's pregnant. Your breasts start to hurt just as when you are pregnant and you retain water.

Some time in your thirties and forties it is likely that the balance between estrogen and progesterone will shift heavily toward estrogen. This excess estrogen (estrogen dominance) is to blame for PMS, night sweats, and depression.

## BREAST CANCER RISK INCREASES IN PERIMENOPAUSE

I wish I had known to listen to the language of my body during perimenopause. I had all the signals. I was the classic example of estrogen dominance. I was moody and bitchy around the house, and I felt justified about being so cranky. The hormonal environment that comes with this dominance is more serious than moodiness, though. This scenario can trigger fetal oncogenes to start flipping on and these oncogenes can contribute to the production of a cancer. This leaves the perimenopausal woman stranded with no source of progesterone to give the signal to turn those cells off because they don't have enough estrogen to "peak" in order to ovulate anymore and there's no placenta on board. Without adequate progesterone, the low chronic estrogen is never turned off, so now the state she is in is life threatening because it can become the backdrop for cancer.

Take perimenopause seriously! Don't ignore your symptoms.

Had I known and understood my symptoms I might have been able to avoid breast cancer. My balance was off. The body likes to be in balance; that's when everything works well. Balance is health and quality of life. Progesterone and estrogen are meant to work together to maintain hormonal *balance* in the body. As your progesterone production diminishes, your quality of life diminishes. Soon your abilities to make estrogen will begin to diminish, and then your symptoms of withdrawal will increase exponentially.

We've all seen what addicts go through when they are withdrawing from their feel-good addictions. Losing our life-giving, youth-giving hormones is a major form of withdrawal and that is why you feel so bad when you enter perimenopause.

The correct ratios between estrogen and progesterone are key. These two hormones are meant to work together to maintain hormone balance. Without balance come mood swings, weight gain, and other even more serious symptoms. Women who have had a hysterectomy also need to balance their monthly cycles with progesterone. (It's amazing to me that most mainstream doctors don't know this.)

## PROGESTERONE— A CAUSE OF POSTPARTUM BLUES?

Here's an interesting fact. In childbirth, once the umbilical cord is cut, all the progesterone whooshes out of the mother into the baby. It is different for each woman: some women's bodies start progesterone production almost immediately after giving birth and they are left feeling happy, blissful, and satisfied. Other women's bodies just take longer to rev up again, leaving those moms in a complete state of hormonal imbalance. They are left feeling like they are going crazy inside, which often results in depression and loads of self-blame. (It's referred to as the postpartum blues.) If this rings a bell, remember: it's not you, it's your hormones, and it's fixable with a qualified doctor (go to ForeverHealth .com) who will adjust your progesterone levels.

## Estrogen

Estrogen is one of the most powerful hormones in the human body; it is what makes a woman a woman. It is estrogen that gives women their softness, their curves and breasts, and helps regulate a woman's passage through menstruation, fertility, and menopause. What many people don't know is that both men and women make estrogen. To be a woman, you need high levels of estrogen and low levels of testosterone. To be a man, you need high levels of testosterone and low levels of estrogen.

Estrogen is not a single hormone. It is a group of many separate yet similar estrogen hormones, which for simplicity's sake can be narrowed down to "the big three": estrone, estradiol, and estriol. These are produced in the ovaries, body fat, and other parts of the body and perform the functions we normally attribute to estrogen.

Approximately three hundred different tissues are equipped with estrogen receptors. This means that estrogen can affect a wide range of tissues and organs, including the brain, liver, bones, and skin. The uterus, urinary tract, breasts, and blood vessels also depend upon estrogen to stay toned and flexible. (Have you ever laughed so hard you peed your pants? Is this happening regularly now? It's because of the estrogen loss that comes with this transition.) Estrogen works in concert with progesterone to nourish and support the growth and regeneration of the female reproductive tissues—breasts, ovaries, and the uterus—so the body will create eggs. In addition, estrogen imparts the characteristic female growth of body hair and its distribution of body fat. It can also protect heart and brain function, and promote bone strength.

*Too Little Estrogen*
Symptoms of estrogen deficiency include:

- Unexplained weight gain
- Apple- or pear-shaped body
- Bloating
- Itching
- Sweating and hot flashes
- Depression
- Irritability
- Weepiness
- Trouble sleeping

- Foggy thinking
- Bladder infections
- Incontinence
- Watery eyes
- Allergies
- Low libido
- Heart palpitations
- Fatigue
- Low bone density
- Painful intercourse

Nice huh? Now are you getting why you aren't feeling so hot?

When a woman is hormonally imbalanced, the body ceases to operate at peak, but the effect is slow and insidious. That's why it takes so long to connect the dots and understand that these symptoms are perimenopausal.

*Excess Estrogen*

But imbalance doesn't only come from producing less, you can also have excess estrogen circulating. Its symptoms include:

- Acne
- Polycystic ovary syndrome (PCOS)
- Infertility
- Ovarian cysts
- Midcycle pain
- Puffiness and bloating
- Cervical dysplasia (abnormal pap smear)
- Rapid weight gain
- Breast tenderness
- Mood swings
- Heavy bleeding
- Anxious depression

- Migraine headaches
- Insomnia
- Foggy thinking
- Red flush on face
- Gallbladder problems
- Weepiness

Estrogen excess leads to a dangerous scenario of building more and more lining within the endometrium (uterus lining) until it becomes so thick you experience breakthrough bleeding, sometimes even hemorrhaging. If this bleeding occurs with frequency, a traditional doctor may recommend a hysterectomy to stop the bleeding. This, frankly, makes my blood boil. We have our body parts for a reason, and to be so cavalier as to remove the uterus as a way to stop bleeding is dangerous, upsetting to the woman, and not very creative. My experts and research tell me that a better remedy for breakthrough bleeding is bioidentical hormone replacement therapy (BHRT) so as to cycle the right amounts of estrogen and progesterone into a woman's body.

Estrogen dominance is a dangerous state. I began to grow my relatively large cancerous breast tumor during perimenopause due to estrogen dominance. (I didn't know enough to go to a doctor for hormones. It just wasn't on the radar at that time.) The problem with a tumor is you can't feel it. Knowing what I know now, I would realize that the puffiness, bloating, mood swings, sleeplessness, and the profuse and frequent breakthrough bleeding (at the time I only felt comfortable wearing black) were indeed symptoms that undiagnosed had profound consequences for me.

It's important to understand that it's imbalanced hormones that have the potential to give cancer cells an opportunity to proliferate.

Symptoms of *estrogen dominance* develop when you don't have enough progesterone to balance the effects of estrogen. Most often, *estrogen excess* or *dominance* is usually reported by women who have declining hormones, are not on any hormone replacement whatsoever, or those taking synthetic hormones or birth control pills. Those symptoms indicate that you are either estrogen dominant or progesterone deficient. In many cases the symptoms are the same. That's why replacing hormones correctly truly is an "art" form. It takes a qualified doctor, doing what is best described as detective work, to find the perfect balance or as I call it "the sweet spot" with natural hormone replacement.

## Testosterone

Testosterone is a naturally occurring anabolic steroid hormone, which means it builds bone and muscle. Your levels always decline around the end of your reproductive years, whether you are male or female. It is an androgen (male hormone), but women also have it. Many don't know that testosterone is very important in relation to the behavior and the general look of a woman. Testosterone is produced in the ovaries and the adrenal glands. Its main function is to provide sex drive; it directly affects sexual sensitivity, clitoris size (and sensitivity), nipple sensitivity, and orgasm. (Pretty nice benefits!)

To limit this important hormone to sex drive alone, though, would be underrating its value. It has many other functions: it maintains bone density, affects muscle size and strength, and is responsible for skin oil secretion.

Testosterone is essential to a woman's hormonal song, although in lower amounts than in men. Testosterone can help with the symptoms of hormonal loss, such as hot flashes and vaginal dryness. It lessens the risk of osteoporosis by improving bone density, reduces body fat, improves mood and lessens depression, improves muscle mass, decreases the risk of autoimmune disorders, fights fatigue, improves symptoms of diabetes, reduces the risk of heart disease, and helps in the treatment of lupus.

Testosterone is essential for a strong working heart. The heart is the largest muscle in the body with more testosterone receptor sites than any other muscle. It is your "pumping power"; testosterone keeps your heart strong.

When you are young, you don't think about your heart much; it's just a given. But ten or twenty years from now you are really going to appreciate having a heart that pumps freely and efficiently. It's about energy and vitality, and the difference between youth and old age is vitality.

Testosterone supports the brain by increasing blood supply and increasing the connections between neurons. It increases the potency of your memory, normalizes your mood, and reduces anxiety.

Testosterone can also make you feel and behave in a more assertive fashion. So many women have had assertiveness programmed out of them, told that "It's not feminine." But this is a tough world, and we are expected to provide for our families in ways never required before. Assertiveness in females is a good thing, but the benefits of testosterone go way beyond this fact.

Perimenopausal women complain of fatigue, aching joints, and a lack of motivation and stamina. Testosterone-deficient women also complain that they feel flabby, and that they are losing muscle tone. I bet you didn't know that women need testosterone to function at their prime, did you? Women can suffer from too much testosterone, as well. Often this imbalance can be caused by consuming too much sugar and eating carbohydrates in excess. Some symptoms of excess testosterone in women include:

- Acne
- High blood pressure

- Excessive hair on face (especially chin) and arms
- Deepened voice
- Polycystic ovary syndrome (PCOS)
- Unstable blood sugar
- Pain when ovulating
- Infertility
- Ovarian cysts

A woman with low testosterone will be more passive and less inclined to do physical activity. This results in abdominal fat, weight gain, lack of self-esteem, lack of confidence, cellulite, varicose veins, and fat accumulation in the breasts, abdomen, and hips. Taking birth control pills (BCPs) will lower the testosterone levels in any woman. If a woman is borderline low, taking BCPs could change her mood, energy, and outlook dramatically. Her look will actually change: she can develop a round back and forward hunching shoulders.

Testosterone in a woman is produced in the ovaries and in the adrenal gland, where DHEA is transformed into testosterone. When you take BCPs, the ovaries take a "rest," which lowers testosterone. Then the woman depends more on the adrenal production and DHEA for her testosterone, yet often this is not enough to do the job.

Testosterone is your friend. It protects against obesity and diabetes by reducing fat mass. It increases lean muscle mass, so you will get more out of your workouts, especially if you are using free weights.

Testosterone is part of the hormonal song. When you were younger and all was working at optimum, you made the right amount of all hormones. When you are ready, your qualified doctor will know through your symptoms and your labs how to produce the perfect alchemy for your individual body.

## DHEA

DHEA is abundantly produced in healthy young adults, but this hormone's levels decline dramatically with advancing age, coinciding with the onset of numerous diseases of aging. DHEA is made by the adrenal glands and converted into testosterone. It is the most plentiful hormone in your body. DHEA is involved in critical body functions and helps support mood, sexual desire, bone density, and a healthy body weight. It has positive effects on the brain, immune system, reproductive organs, muscles, and other organs and tissues. It has effects ranging from prevention of heart disease and cancer to the promotion of weight loss. DHEA also helps to maintain collagen levels in the skin, promoting smooth, young-looking skin.

French scientists studied the effects of DHEA replacement therapy in about three hundred men and women between the ages of sixty and eighty over the course of a year. One of the findings to come out of this well-known study (known as the DHEAge study) was that DHEA supplementation greatly improved the color, tone, thickness, and hydration of the subjects' skin (*see* University of Maryland Medical Center). DHEA is known as *the* antiaging hormone.

It is important that perimenopausal women understand DHEA, and not just because of its skin benefits. This hormone peaks between the ages of twenty-three and thirty and then begins to drop off. By the time you are fifty you have only a fraction of the DHEA you had in your late twenties. This drop-off parallels the general decline in your health and vitality as you age. Stress accelerates the natural decline of DHEA levels.

What's interesting about DHEA is that it can help the levels of other sex hormones, thus providing many women with the boost they need to replace hormones slowly being lost to aging. Recent scientific evidence confirms that restoring DHEA to youthful levels may help safely boost estrogen and testosterone levels by a small amount (*see* University of Maryland Medical Center and its supporting research). Bonus: this one is affordable for everyone and the benefits are far-reaching. It is one of the few "legal" hormones you can purchase with or without a prescription.

DHEA is a relatively unknown hormone to the general population, yet it is remarkable in all aspects of its effectiveness. I asked Bill Faloon, the founder of the Life Extension Foundation, a nonprofit organization over thirty-three years old dedicated to health and well-being, to share with me some of his organization's research on DHEA. Life Extension is responsible for bringing this hormone to the United States and making it legal, which was no easy feat. The information that follows encapsulates the highlights of what he told me.

There are many studies that substantiate the benefits of DHEA. Research supports DHEA's critical role in:

- Alleviating depression
- Preventing atherosclerosis
- Increasing bone mass
- Slowing osteoporosis
- Improving insulin resistance
- Hastening wound healing

In perimenopausal women, normal DHEA levels stimulate adequate production of a substance called insulin-like growth factor 1 (IGF-1), which maintains new bone formation. Healthy DHEA levels also suppress production of interleukin-6, an inflammatory cytokine that causes excessive bone breakdown. DHEA's suppression of interleukin-6 helps prevent bone loss and chronic inflammatory disorders.

Perimenopausal and older women should monitor their levels through annual blood testing (you can test more often if needed). Your objective is to be on the high side of normal, which for women is between 250 and 380 ug/dL of blood.

If DHEA blood levels are below the optimal range, this tells you it's time to begin supplementation. After three to six weeks of DHEA supplementation, a blood test is suggested to assess DHEA levels and adjust dosage. Individuals with existing hormone-sensitive cancers should talk with their doctors before using DHEA. With proper monitoring DHEA replacement therapy is a very safe and extraordinarily effective antiaging therapy for most people. Individuals with cancer, though, are an area of potential concern. This is why the use of any hormone should be monitored by a qualified doctor.

## Oxytocin—the Sex/Love Hormone

Often as we experience hormonal decline we not only suffer from estrogen deficiency but also become deficient in oxytocin. Estrogen has profound effects upon oxytocin in the brain (see McCarthy). When this happens, you experience a feeling of being cut off from others; it's an isolated, lonely feeling.

Oxytocin is one of the newer discovered hormones, the "cuddle" hormone that we associate with pregnancy. It is given to women during childbirth to induce labor. It also is produced by nursing mothers, which helps during this busy and amazing time to allow a mom to relax and feel loving toward her child rather than stressed. According to Dr. Prudence Hall, my gynecologist (who wrote the foreword for this book), "Oxytocin causes people to feel natural happiness and love and reduces anxiety; it also causes women to feel more orgasmic."

Now, I've got your attention.

Supplementing with oxytocin allows women to experience

better and stronger orgasms. This is a very important hormone for perimenopausal women to consider, many of whom are stressed over the new inability to *feel* sex. Oxytocin causes better arousal so it's one of the important sexual and social hormones.

We are sexual and social animals who naturally want to bond with other people, and this hormone helps you connect and relax. Oxytocin also helps you lose weight because it curbs appetite, while giving you a sense of well-being. Good-bye stress eating.

A nursing mother releases tremendous amounts of oxytocin with no side effects, so for a nonnursing woman, especially a woman in hormonal decline, this is a delicious addition to consider adding to your hormonal repertoire. Everything about it is good: it helps you maintain a sense of inner peace, and it decreases the feeling of pain in the body. It also helps with insomnia and your general feeling of vitality, plus . . . it makes you want to have a lot of sex.

### Pregnenolone

Pregnenolone is made by the adrenals and is a little-known sexual stimulant. Pregnenolone supplementation on a daily basis increases sexual arousal and promotes better orgasm. This hormone also protects our brains and keeps our memories sharp. It gives energy, vitality, and did I mention a better sex drive? Pregnenolone is important for weight loss. When the adrenals are low due to stress, it's very common to find that pregnenolone levels are low too.

Pregnenolone is a "mother hormone" because it helps to make a lot of other hormones in the body. Doctors use pregnenolone to bring low progesterone up to target levels, because it gently boosts low progesterone. This in turn will also correct progesterone/estrogen ratios.

Pregnenolone is also referred to as the "memory hormone."

In animal studies it improves memory one hundred times more than DHEA in the same dose. It enhances memory at least in part because it is believed to help clarify thinking and stimulate concentration. At higher doses it has been shown to reduce fatigue, fight depression, protect the joints, relieve arthritis, and speed healing.

Without enough pregnenolone you are sure to have memory problems and poor concentration. Without it you'll be vulnerable to stress and depression and at risk for chronic fatigue and reduced capacity for physical exertion. Because pregnenolone feeds production of so many other hormones, if you don't have sufficient levels of this one, you'll create a domino effect with the others, creating a host of other symptoms. For example, you might get slack muscles and lack of hair under your arms and in the pubic area, which generally signifies low DHEA or low blood pressure, and the weight loss that is linked to low cortisol levels. Low blood pressure and dizzy spells when standing up are related to insufficient aldosterone and will be affected by a lack of sufficient pregnenolone.

Pregnenolone is available over the counter. Interestingly, it is made from cholesterol by mitochondria (the energy center of each cell in our body) and is the compound within cells from which DHEA, progesterone, estrogen, cortisol, and testosterone are created. As I've said above, pregnenolone increases brain activity. Those who have problems learning or remembering may benefit from supplementation.

It's clear to me that nature worked it all out. Now our job is to replicate the perfection of nature as best we can by putting back that which is missing to make our bodies operate at peak.

Okay, we've covered the minor hormones, now let's go to the majors . . .

# CHAPTER 4

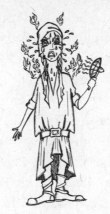

# THE MAJOR HORMONES—
# AND THE IMPORTANCE OF BALANCE

Male andropause is a lot more fun than female perimenopause. With female perimenopause you gain weight and get hot flashes. Male andropause—you get to date young girls and drive motorcycles.

—Unknown author

At this point, you want relief and you are anxious to get to it. Now that you understand the vital role of your minor hormones, it's time to learn the important functions of the major hormones. After all, it's hard to properly fix what you don't fully understand.

The major hormones—insulin, thyroid, adrenaline, and cortisol—are the first to be secreted in response to our constantly changing nutrition, lifestyle, and environmental signals. The majors are crucial for life-sustaining functions such as regulating heartbeat and blood pressure, and also for maintaining the pH balance between blood acidity and alkalinity.

The major and minor hormones communicate with each other, but the major hormones have greater influence on the body and in the hormonal "discussion." If a major hormone is not replaced, you will die rather quickly; they are that important and crucial to life. With the loss of a minor hormone, you will not feel well, but you are likely to attribute your poor health to normal aging and not seek medical attention. You will eventually die from the loss of minor hormones, but it may be ten to fifty years later. At that point no one will attribute your death to loss of hormones: they'll call it cancer, or Alzheimer's, or heart attack.

If any of these major hormones are low or missing, there is no question about whether or not to replace them. You would never deny a diabetic his regular injections of insulin. Insulin keeps the diabetic alive. Let's begin by understanding the role of each individual MAJOR hormone.

First I'd like to give you a visual:

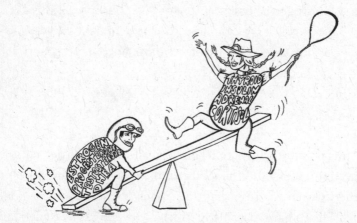

Imagine an old-fashioned teeter-totter that you may have played on as a kid at the park or playground.

But instead of your best friend sitting there and holding you up in the air, on one end are the *minor hormones:* estrogen, progesterone, testosterone, DHEA (pregnenolone and oxytocin are also minors but they are secondary hormones).

On the other end of the teeter-totter are the *major hormones:* thyroid, insulin, adrenaline, and cortisol.

When you start to "dip" in the minor hormones (which are indicated by the symptoms you are beginning to feel), the other end of the teeter-totter rises.

Minors get low—you get symptomatic; majors rise—you get symptomatic. With insulin high (because your minors are low), you can't lose weight. You can't lose weight if your thyroid is off, either. If your cortisol and adrenaline are high, because one of the minors is low, you can't sleep.

Result: you are a mess!

In traditional medicine, because there is still a tremendous lack of understanding regarding hormonal decline and imbalance, you may be given medication to suppress these symptoms: sleeping pills, antidepressants, diuretics, diet medications, if not more. In almost all cases, these are unnecessary and even can be dangerous. With an understanding of each of these major hormones you will be able to read and evaluate your personal body "language" to fight back using the appropriate, non-drug remedies to get to the true root of your hormone-related problems.

Let's talk insulin. Why do we need to? Because it's a fat-storing hormone. Got your attention, again, didn't I? Good. Read on.

### Insulin

Insulin has many functions in the body. It is a major hormone secreted by the islet cells of the pancreas, which helps to move glucose from the blood into the cells for use as energy. Insulin determines whether nutrients taken in will be burned off as energy or stored as fat. This is why insulin is called the *fat-storing hormone*.

You don't want high insulin. Insulin resistance is a result of high insulin levels. How do you get high insulin? Since our hormones are all interconnected, the teeter-totter visual is most effective for explaining it. When the minor hormones dip, as they do during perimenopause, your insulin levels go higher. Estrogen is important in optimizing insulin response in the cells.

High insulin tends to impede the release of other hormones involved in the body's ability to burn stored body fat. A pattern of high levels of glucose and insulin in the bloodstream will cause glucose to be stored as fat. Insulin resistance is also a precursor to type 2 diabetes.

Here's how insulin resistance develops. Normally, glucose (or blood sugar) goes up after eating; insulin is then produced so we can utilize the glucose to be used by muscle or stored as fat. The insulin level is then supposed to drop quickly to its normal low level. As we get older and have less estrogen and more body fat, our insulin receptors become less functional and the body can't handle glucose as effectively. When the brain detects continued high glucose levels, it signals the pancreas to release even more insulin to lower the blood sugar level. As a result, blood sugar levels plummet, which makes the body ravenous for all the wrong foods to try to bring the blood sugar level up quickly.

Insulin resistance is also exacerbated by high cortisol levels, and this high cortisol can contribute to significant weight gain as well as compromising your immune function and increasing your risk of heart disease (chronic high cortisol often leads to heart attack or stroke).

I've been writing about the insulin phenomenon for years, both in my Somersize books and more recently in my *Sexy For-*

*ever* series. I have advised past readers that to lose weight, they must acquaint themselves not only with the dangers of sugar, but also with food that the body converts to sugar, and then avoid those foods. These foods—white flour, white rice, high-starch vegetables, refined white sugar, and any food that contains sugar—promote insulin secretion. When insulin is secreted, blood sugar rises from eating sugary foods; so you need to avoid these harmful foods, otherwise you will be fighting fat regardless of how much you exercise. So many women your age are experiencing the puzzle that stumps everyone: Why, when you are eating less and working out more, are you gaining weight? Now you know, it's your hormones!

In addition to perimenopause's hormonal decline, there are other factors that can affect insulin levels. Here is a look at the habits and factors that raise insulin:

- Low-fat diets
- Excessive intake of carbohydrates
- Fake food, including: saccharin, aspartame, margarine, and most other invented substances found in overly refined, processed foods
- Consumption of soft drinks
- Overconsumption of alcohol
- Smoking
- Use of recreational stimulants
- Stress
- Lack of exercise
- Some types of prescription drugs (particularly antidepressants; they calm you down but slow your metabolism at the same time—there's no free lunch)
- Steroids, which have a tendency to make the face and body puffy
- Diet pills

If you continue with a high-insulin style of eating or the lifestyle habits that help spike insulin, both your immune and hormone systems will age faster. Prolonged high insulin levels are one of the leading causes of accelerated metabolic aging.

Understanding that high insulin levels are caused in large part by declining hormones will help you to understand why your body is changing and how you can get it back. Take insulin levels seriously; watch your diet, exercise and balance your hormones, and you will be able to delay and most probably eliminate high insulin, adding another reason to enjoy your perimenopausal experience.

## Cravings—Why Are You Experiencing More Now?

It's important to understand the estrogen connection to high insulin levels. When estrogen levels are low, we crave carbohydrates. This is why women frequently comb the cupboards for chocolate right before their periods when their estrogen levels are at their lowest. A low estrogen state makes it impossible for a woman to avoid carbohydrate craving, since estrogen is one of the hormones necessary for serotonin production (the feel-good brain neurotransmitter). When she gives in and consumes the sugar, chocolates, or carbohydrates, her insulin levels shoot up. Her brain gets the dopamine "hit" it needs, but now she craves more sugar and carbohydrates and the merry-go-round begins. (For more on what to do when a chocolate craving hits go to The Symptom Solver, pages 211 and 212.) You are going to get off that merry-go-round and to a place of feeling great without the chocolate hit. (That doesn't mean I'm saying no to chocolate! But you want your brain happy without outside crutches.)

I'm telling you again . . . this passage isn't for sissies!

## Thyroid

The thyroid is a butterfly-shaped gland located in the lower part of the neck just below the Adam's apple. It has many functions and is a major player in your feeling of well-being. It is amazing how many aspects of the body are affected by this one small but very significant gland. Our metabolic rate is driven by the thyroid; that fact is well known. But you might not know that the thyroid can also impact blood pressure, breathing, digestion, and nerve function.

The thyroid affects virtually every system in your body. The human body is composed of approximately sixty to ninety trillion cells. All cells communicate with one another and every cell in the body is affected by the thyroid because it regulates the rate at which energy is consumed by the cells. (Remember the teeter-totter, when the minors go low the majors rise or even turn off?) Well, in perimenopause, low estrogen and/or low progesterone can leave you with either a slowed or an overactive thyroid.

To understand unexplained weight gain, fibrocystic breasts, joint pain, hair loss, loss of sex drive, and so many other complaints, then you need to understand the thyroid—which is why you'll notice that this section of the chapter is longer than for the other majors. It's that important. If your thyroid isn't "right," then you won't feel "right." It's that simple.

The thyroid, along with the adrenals, is the gland most susceptible to malfunction in our fast-paced, stressed lifestyles. Yet correcting a thyroid condition, perhaps more than any other of the major hormones, is an art. The more you understand how it works, the greater the chance you can achieve lifelong balance with all your hormones. On a cellular level, there can be no optimal nutrition absorption, detoxification of wastes, or stimulation of oxygen consumption without thyroid balance.

If your thyroid is out of whack, it can produce too much or too little of the hormone. Since we're looking, like Goldilocks, for "just right," you want neither state. Not too high, not too low, just right.

## THYROID: A PEEK UNDER THE HOOD

The thyroid secretes iodine-containing hormones, triiodothyronine (T3) and thyroxine (T4), which regulate body temperature, heart rate, and metabolism. The thyroid works by taking orders from the pituitary gland and the hypothalamus, which are constantly monitoring the amount of thyroxine (T4) circulating in the blood. When the level of thyroxine gets low, the pituitary gland releases thyroid-stimulating hormone (TSH). As the name suggests, thyroid-stimulating hormone signals the thyroid to produce more thyroxine (T4). As the amount of thyroxine in the blood increases, the production of TSH is suppressed. This in turn slows the production of thyroxine. This feedback loop between the pituitary and thyroid works to keep the level of thyroid hormone relatively constant in the body.

Once in the body, circulating T4 is converted to the active form of T3. As we age, the production of T4 diminishes. In addition, the conversion of T4 to T3 also diminishes, resulting in less information being transferred from cell to cell. Now your body is not working at maximum. The information pathway is being interrupted and symptoms begin to reveal themselves.

Here we go again; when the minors dip, your body has trouble converting T4 to T3, and hypothyroidism (low or underactive thyroid) occurs. Overweight women with a family history of obesity may have lower levels of T3 in their blood. Treatments to raise T3 levels may help reduce some metabolic risk factors associated with abdominal obesity in some of these overweight women.

Now here is where many doctors don't get it right. They test thyroid for T4 only. T4 can come back in normal ranges, even though you are displaying all symptoms of low thyroid. You have to insist your doctor test for T4 *and* T3. Without reviewing free T3 levels you will not get an accurate reading and your symptoms (from mild to severe) will continue.

## Hyperthyroidism

In *hyperthyroidism,* or Graves' disease, your thyroid becomes overactive and produces too much thyroid. You can usually tell by looking at a person whose body is in this state, as a symptom of it is slightly bulging eyeballs.

Too much thyroid can damage your cells, particularly those in your heart and other muscles. It can also increase your risk of osteoporosis. With hyperthyroidism, your body's metabolism is set too high and gaining weight becomes difficult. You become tired at the end of the day but then feel wired, agitated, and unable to sleep. Your hands might tremble and you may find yourself being easily upset. Diarrhea is common in hyperthyroidism, as is nervousness and warm, moist, coarse, and/or red skin, particularly on the shins.

If your hyperthyroidism is severe, your doctor might prescribe antithyroid medications to slow down its production, or he or she may even suggest thyroid ablation. Thyroid ablation is a procedure that requires surgery or the use of radioactive iodine to destroy much, if not all, of your thyroid with radioactive iodine or surgery. My feeling is these treatments can create other problems. Knowing that the thyroid is so vital to health and quality of life, I would think radioactive thyroid ablation should be the very last resort. Without a thyroid gland, it will require an amazing doctor to constantly monitor and adjust thyroid replacement.

With age and stress, hormones need adjusting so it seems like it would be better to first try and lower your thyroid naturally through diet and hormone replacement, with the help of a qualified doctor.

## Hypothyroidism

In contrast, someone with a condition of hypothyroidism produces too little thyroid hormone. This, the most common thyroid disorder, typically strikes after age forty, which is perimenopause's prime time. Low thyroid is generally misunderstood and is often left underdiagnosed and undertreated, which can lead to a host of issues. Untreated thyroid disease has been tied to elevated cholesterol levels, heart disease, infertility, fatigue, muscle weakness, poor mental function, depression, weight gain, and an increased risk of cancer. Without the intervention of a qualified doctor, the older you get, the more likely your thyroid function is going to slow down. Endocrinologists estimate that one in five women and one in ten men over sixty suffer from underactive thyroids. .

Your thyroid can become low or underactive as a result of a genetic inheritance, exposure to certain viruses, iodine deficiency, direct physical trauma to the thyroid, indirect trauma (such as whiplash), autoimmune disease, or environmental toxins. In some cases the body itself will produce thyroid antibodies in a mistaken immune response, where the body perceives it is under threat and then produces antibodies to attack and disarm the threat. Insufficient dietary iodine can also cause hypothyroidism (as well as fibrocystic breasts). Iodine is utilized by every hormone receptor in the body, so deficient iodine can result in problems such as ovarian cysts, thyroid goiters, and hormonal imbalances.

Low thyroid causes weight gain. It is a classic symptom of this dysfunction. In such cases, levels of thyroid-stimulating hormone (TSH) may rise in an attempt to spur more production and secretion of thyroid hormones from the thyroid gland. Other symptoms include: cold intolerance, particularly the extremities (cold hands and feet), fatigue, dry skin and follicular keratosis (like goose bumps on the triceps' skin on the back of the arm), constipation, obesity/difficulty losing weight, swelling all over (swollen eyelids, swollen calves), hoarse morning voice, morning depression, orange coloration on the soles of the feet, slow pulse rate, high diastolic blood pressure, slow Achilles tendon reflexes, slow thinking, poor concentration, muscle and articular pains, PMS, menstrual abnormalities, low libido, brittle nails, frequent colds, flu, and other infections. As you can see from this long list of symptoms, low thyroid is no joke.

Depression is also frighteningly common. Many women with thyroid problems suffer from depression. One explanation for this is that T3 is actually a neurotransmitter that regulates the action of serotonin (the feel-good hormone) and norepinephrine, two brain chemicals that are important for alleviating depression (*see* Mason; Sintzel).

Perhaps the most awful of all symptoms, and this one is not common, is losing control of *you* and acting irrationally, crazy, literally out of control. It can begin as low-grade depression, but in severe cases people can experience hallucinations and delusions. This rare condition is sometimes referred to as "hypothyroid insanity." Other symptoms of it are mental confusion, loss of memory, and delusions of persecution. I often wonder if those who go on shooting rampages are delusional from low thyroid. It is certainly something to consider. I mention it only because in the extreme chance that you recognize yourself in this description, you should immediately contact a doctor for help.

## Hashimoto's Thyroiditis

Hashimoto's is another form of dysfunctional thyroid, though not common, that women write to me about. It is a condition that causes the body's defenses, the immune system, to produce antibodies that over time destroy thyroid tissue. As a result, the thyroid gland cannot make enough thyroid hormone. The inflammation of the thyroid that results from the body's attack is aggravated by food allergies and intolerances (usually gluten, wheat, and other grains; and sweets, even including fruits like grapes or dried fruit). Hashimoto's disease is complex, but its symptoms are worth recognizing. They may be mild at first or take years to develop. The first sign of the disease is often an enlarged thyroid, called a goiter. The goiter may cause the front of your neck to look swollen. A large goiter may make swallowing difficult. Other symptoms of an underactive thyroid due to Hashimoto's disease may include: unexplained weight gain, fatigue, paleness or puffiness of the face, joint and muscle pain, constipation, inability to get warm, difficulty getting pregnant, hair loss or thinning/brittleness, irregular or heavy menstrual periods, depression, and slowed heart rate.

There is no cure for Hashimoto's disease, but don't despair. There is no "cure" for perimenopause either, but we know now that by putting back the hormones you are missing you can regain your quality of life. With Hashimoto's disease, replacing thyroid correctly and regulating iodine can balance hormone levels.

## The New Normal—Optimal Thyroid Ranges

Thyroid function tests tell you whether your thyroid is working normally. Your symptoms will also tell you, if you are in tune with the language of your body. When TSH is measured, most doctors consider normal to be in the 0.2 to 5.5 range. However, the normal range is no longer considered optimal by antiaging doctors. Optimal is between 1.0 and 2.0; higher than this and you can experience premature aging and an increased risk of heart disease. Philip Miller, M.D., author of *The Life Extension Revolution*, says, "If your thyroid levels are above 4.0 (still considered normal range), you are at increased risk of heart disease."

You may be going to a doctor with complaints that indicate your thyroid is too high or too low, but then your blood work comes back in the normal range. Your doctor therefore, may not treat your thyroid because he or she considers it normal. Yet it could be one of the big reasons you are symptomatic and gaining weight. When the thyroid is not working at optimal range for *you*, you will not get the full benefit of bioidentical hormone replacement therapy, should you choose to use it.

The thyroid is very complex, and it takes a master to understand and interpret your labs fully. That is why you need to know the symptoms and tell your doctor everything that you are feeling. Hypothyroidism is very common in perimenopause, as I stated earlier, because estrogen and progesterone levels become imbalanced. Your ovaries have thyroid receptors on them and your thyroid gland has ovarian receptors (see how they interact with one another?). When your ovaries stop making estrogen, your thyroid is also affected.

Whenever thyroid problems are suspected or treated, it is important to monitor adrenal function as well. Attempting to treat low thyroid levels without supporting the adrenals can deplete the adrenal glands. At the same time, if your adrenals are weak, symptoms of low thyroid may persist even after your thyroid levels have been restored. Let's find out more about the adrenal glands.

## Adrenaline

Adrenal fatigue is a collection of signs and symptoms that results from low function of the adrenal glands. The paramount symptom is fatigue that is not relieved by sleep. The syndrome may be caused by intense or prolonged stress, or after acute or chronic infections, especially respiratory infections such as influenza, bronchitis, or pneumonia . . . people suffering from adrenal fatigue often have to use coffee, colas, and other stimulants to get going in the morning and to prop themselves up during the day.

—James L. Wilson, *Adrenal Fatigue*

I like to describe the hormones of the body as a symphony. The *adrenals* are the conductor. Adrenaline comes from two triangular glands, the adrenals, which sit on top of each kidney. The adrenals also produce cortisol and together with adrenaline speed up heart rate, regulate blood pressure, and aid in other bodily functions that help you cope with stress. We'll get to cortisol in a bit; for now I want to focus on adrenaline.

The adrenals' hormones are also (like the thyroid) directed by the hypothalamus, which then communicate with the pituitary. The pituitary in turn communicates with the thyroid and then back to the adrenals. In this loop, the adrenals communicate with all the other hormones, telling them what to do. If all the hormones are balanced and in perfect working order, the symphony is in tune. It is *harmonic*. We all know how beautiful that sounds. It's the same with the body. When all is in perfect tune, you feel in harmony. You feel wonderful. If the orchestra leader (adrenals) doesn't show up, then all the other players who are able to play don't know *what* to play, so they become discordant. Sadly, most people are not in tune; they have no harmony. That is why aging becomes accelerated. Most people are walking around feeling unwell. Because they are not flat-out sick (yet) they accept it as the way it is. They don't know that having hormonal harmony creates a state of bliss.

It is important to your quality of life that all your hormones are working at optimum. This is why I am spending so much time in this chapter dissecting each hormone's function and purpose.

Adrenaline is our engine . . . it pushes us forward. You've felt it, that surge of boundless energy. If we are living a balanced life, our bodies release adrenaline when we need that surge and then afterward we return to a calmer baseline.

Problems arise when we get addicted to adrenaline and put ourselves in situations that continually feed our bodies more and more of it. These people are "adrenaline junkies." You don't need to be jumping out of airplanes to be addicted to adrenaline. You just need to be "on" at all times, craving or living in a high-energy state nonstop. You know these people; you may be one of them: every minute of each day is filled with activities, responsibilities, and piles and piles of things on the to-do list, with lots of check marks ticking off completed tasks. It is often said, "If you want something done fast and well, ask the busiest person you know." There is truth in that statement. These busy, busy people are likely running on adrenaline, nature's best energy bar. But like a caffeine bump or an illicit drug's high, it's addictive and also dangerous to your health.

Why is it a problem? Because if you continue down this path you can "blow out" your adrenals and they can become fatigued. Once that happens your adrenals won't produce enough cortisol, and it will go too low. I know firsthand; I've blown out my adrenals from overwork and overbusyness, myself. It's not fun!

When your adrenals are burned out the way mine were, you have no energy and you feel a "racing" inside that makes sleep impossible, which further hurts the function of your adrenals. The lack of sleep makes everything worse. What do you do when you are exhausted? You crave caffeine, or drugs, any stimulant that gives a false sense of energy. When you don't sleep soundly for days, weeks, even months (or like me, *three years!*), the result is depression.

The sad thing is most women go to their doctors at this point and instead of understanding the major impact of burned-out adrenals, their doctors will give them antidepressants like Paxil or Prozac. Now you are in trouble. Resorting to these substances is a road to nowhere, leaving you in a worse state.

I have burned out my adrenals three times in my career. It feels terrible, and it shortens your life. It also is a setup for a heart attack. I've had a tendency to overwork and reached total burn-out too often. Think about this the next time you find yourself awarded the honor of being the busiest person you know. Who is really benefiting? Certainly not you!

People who have adrenal insufficiency suffer a lot. They are not calm. They live feeling like at any moment the sky is going to fall. They also are generally more negative than others. And, guess what, most of us are in this boat. The American Academy for the Advancement of Medicine (ACAM) estimates that 85 percent of Americans are walking around with burned-out adrenals, meaning adrenal burnout and borderline adrenal burnout are very common. The diagnosis is difficult because the causes are different: it could be from imbalanced minor hormones, over-working (superwoman syndrome), or a high level of toxicity causing you to have great difficulty to operate at maximum, or all of the above.

Other symptoms of adrenal fatigue include:

- Exhaustion
- Heart palpitations
- Recurrent infections
- Achiness
- Low blood sugar
- Inability to sleep

In addition to overwork and busyness, here are some of the other factors that can cause it:

- Anemia
- Not enough rest, sleeplessness
- Hormone imbalance
- Inflammation
- Infections
- Dietary imbalances
- Poor diet with excess calories from junk food
- Birth control pills
- Overexercising

See yourself in this list?

The correction for burned-out adrenals includes sleep, a change in your diet, and a shift in your thinking. The present situation is not serving you well, so it's time to change.

I vowed never to do that to myself again. I changed my life. I reprioritized my daily schedule, made time for sleep. I do yoga three times a week, and I realize that relaxation time is as important as being busy. I no longer stay up late, whereas I used to stay up until the wee hours of the morning writing my books. Now I try to be in bed by 9:00 p.m. It takes retraining. I have readjusted my social schedule so that I do not go out two nights in a row, and I try not to go out more than two nights a week. I know had I not done this, I would be in big trouble by now.

Your doctor can test for adrenal fatigue with a simple saliva test to determine if your adrenals are blown out. These same tests also measure your cortisol levels. Whether you are producing too much or too little cortisol, adrenal imbalance can lead to serious health problems . . . which is why the next major hormone you need to know more about is cortisol.

## Cortisol

Cortisol is your stress hormone. It is released by your adrenal glands. When you encounter a stressful situation, you quickly release cortisol to raise your blood sugar level and give you energy. You've heard of those instances where a five-foot-nothing mom lifts a car to save her trapped child? Well, that's cortisol at work mobilizing energy and fast. It's the same as if you were to encounter a knife-wielding stranger. Your body springs into action, thanks to adrenaline and cortisol, so you can quickly run away. Crazy events like this aside, you cannot live very long without cortisol. It is that important to your body's functioning.

Cortisol is the only major hormone where if you do not have any of it, you will die at the first body stressor, like an infection. (I told you it was important.) Cortisol is needed for mood enhancement, dynamism, work capacity, stress resistance, stimulation of our immune defenses, antirheumatic action (joint pains), and antipain action.

If cortisol production is too low, you will have symptoms, such as fatigue, muscle weakness, sweating, mood changes like anxiety and depression, and muscle and joint pain, plus an inability to have control over emotions leaving you feeling sharp and more prone to verbal retorts, nervousness, and irritability.

Your body will secrete cortisol for whatever stress you encounter, including: a bad day at work, a near miss in the car, stressing over a missed deadline, or a death in the family. It doesn't differentiate the stressor; it just pours out the hormone. Stress raises your blood pressure and uses up your energy reserves without much benefit to you. Using up your stores by stressing on the "small stuff" is a waste. With no threat to your life, you're using up hormones that are crucial to your well-being and your longevity. They say we experience more stress in one day in today's world than people of Elizabethan time did in their entire life-times! Stress is a wasted emotion that takes its toll on every part of your body, both emotionally and physically.

## Too High

Symptoms of excess cortisol production are:

- Extra fat around the neck
- Anxiety
- Bloating
- Memory problems
- Irregular periods
- Food cravings
- High blood pressure
- Elevated blood sugar
- Increased appetite
- Insomnia and sleep problems
- Irritability
- Excess hair growth on the body and face
- No libido
- Skin problems, thin skin, bruising
- Weight gain and fat buildup

Also note: chronically elevated cortisol levels will eventually degrade your immune system. This is a dangerous place to be, since you will have difficulty fighting off infections, especially viral infections. Stressed-out people are more susceptible to colds and flus as well as flare-ups of cold sores or shingles. Cancer patients with high cortisol have little ability to fight the cancer, which increases the chances that the cancer will metastasize throughout the body.

The stress connection goes on and on and is even harmful to

your brain cells. It can impair cognitive function, which means your memory, your reaction time, your problem-solving abilities, and your learning abilities. In short, high cortisol ages the brain.

But the most awful damage that can happen from high cortisol is the damage to the heart. If you recall again the teeter-totter: when the minors drop, the majors rise. Chronic *high* cortisol almost always leads to heart disease, heart attack, or stroke (*see* De Leo).

As I said, cortisol is the hormone needed to handle stress. So when under stress, the body in its wisdom will produce more cortisol to handle the difficult situation and less of the other hormones, such as aldosterone, DHEA, and pregnenolone. This is the body adapting, stealing from one to rev up production of another; in this case, the normally high cortisol compensates by going higher, and in turn your production of DHEA goes down.

When DHEA is low, pregnenolone and aldosterone steroid hormones, which are made from cholesterol, are low and the body tries to repair itself by telling the liver to make more cholesterol. Result: high cholesterol and now your health is at further risk. Cholesterol has been made out to be the bad guy, but our body makes cholesterol for many functions; it is responsible for producing cortisol, testosterone, estrogen, DHEA, aldosterone, and pregnenolone. In other words, we need cholesterol in the right amounts.

## Too Low . . . Fatigue and Burnout

The body tries to compensate for all your stress, but at some point it just can't; and when cortisol production becomes too low, the result is adrenal burnout or fatigue, as we discussed in the adrenaline section. This means the adrenals can no longer secrete the levels of cortisol commensurate with the levels of stress.

In the first phase of adrenal fatigue, your body produces enough cortisol for everyday activities, but not enough to handle stressful situations. That's why a big event will leave you all shaken, or a cold or flu can seem to last forever. You are prone to pneumonia, bronchitis, asthma, sinusitis, or respiratory infections (recurrent respiratory infections are almost always a sign of low adrenal function). Now you are in a vicious cycle, like I was, and every stressful situation depletes a little more of your adrenal reserves, causing even lower adrenal function and worsening symptoms.

If your adrenals are burned out, then your hormones will be imbalanced. It's that simple. In perimenopause, your progesterone and estrogen have dropped, which pushes the cortisol high. But with burnout it stays high, so sleep becomes impossible.

## Cortisol and Body Fat

Cortisol is also connected to increased body fat. High levels of cortisol can create insulin resistance. As you know from earlier in this chapter, insulin resistance is a condition in which the cells of the body become resistant to the effects of insulin, and higher levels of insulin are produced by the pancreas. Left unchecked, it can lead to diabetes, and worse. When you are insulin resistant, your body doesn't handle dietary sugars or carbohydrates very well, producing spikes in blood sugar that damage blood vessels.

When your cortisol is chronically elevated because of stress, it creates a devastating cycle of alternating high blood sugar and high insulin. Unchecked insulin resistance can also lead to syndrome X, also known as metabolic syndrome. This condition is characterized by abdominal obesity, high cholesterol, high triglycerides, and high blood pressure.

It's easy to see why perimenopausal women are at risk for this condition when you understand that it is triggered by high cortisol. With lower estrogen and progesterone, we now know, comes higher cortisol.

After a while, your body loses its sensitivity to this cycle of alternating high blood sugar and high insulin, and then the results can be tragic. You can see clearly how the dangerous progression from elevated cortisol to elevated blood sugar to insulin resistance is one of the major ways stress contributes to heart disease, obesity, diabetes, and even death.

A poor diet, not enough sleep, and no exercise can raise cortisol levels. Also, cortisol is made from progesterone, so if your cortisol levels are too high for too long, the "progesterone steal" occurs and your body steals away progesterone to make cortisol. The takeaway: too much stress/cortisol equals too little progesterone.

As I said, I have overworked too many times in my career and have so taxed my adrenals and cortisol levels that I have flatlined and burned out my abilities to make adequate cortisol. Don't be like me. Don't do this to yourself. It was stupid of me, thinking I needed to outwork everyone. We women do that. We will work till we drop. I actually did drop, woke up crying one Christmas morning thinking my life was worthless (cortisol induced). This kind of burnout causes severe depression, and the only remedy is cortisol replacement, vitamin B shots, and sleep, sleep, and more sleep. It takes about a year to normalize burned-out adrenals and cortisol.

You've got all the tools you'll need in this book to help you eliminate stress and save your cortisol reserves for when you really need them, as in life-threatening situations.

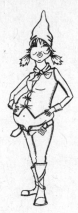

# CHAPTER 5

# WHAT TO EAT AND WHY TO SUPPLEMENT— NUTRIENTS THAT MAKE A BIG DIFFERENCE

In an ideal world we would eat well all the time. Our food would not be grown in nutrient-poor soil that contains pesticides and heavy metals from acid rain. Cattle, chickens, and other animals wouldn't be raised in unsanitary conditions, pumped full of hormones and antibiotics. Produce wouldn't be cleaned and packaged in huge factory-like warehouses where E. coli and other bacteria can quickly spread and become untraceable, an unfortunate by-product of mass production that is known to contaminate even organic food.

—*The Immortality Edge,* by Michael Fossel, MD; Greta Blackburn; and Dave Woynarowski, MD

The air we breathe, the water we drink, and the food we eat determines our health and our quality of life. But sadly, today our air is polluted, our water is filled with contaminants, and our food has essentially been hijacked. In other words, to survive, to achieve peak health with great life quality you are going to have to aggressively change your reality and clean up your environment as well as your body.

Changing how we eat is not a difficult thing to do. If up until now your choices have been less than stellar, changing your ways and making good food choices is crucial. To stay healthy and hormonally balanced, you have to take food seriously. That means ditching the junk food.

## JUNK FOOD

Let's talk about junk food as it pertains to perimenopause. For starters, it is laden with chemicals. There is probably nothing worse you could do to your body, at any time but especially now, than to go out of your way to load it up with toxic chemicals. Your master antioxidant, glutathione, has considerably reduced over the passing years, so the protection afforded you in your first three decades of life is now diminished. Free radicals in the form of junk food start to reside in your intestines, causing bloating, fatigue, and a downgraded immune system. The body, in its wisdom, in trying to keep these toxic chemicals away from your precious organs and glands, does you a favor and stores them in your fat. The more toxins (fast food, junk food, pesticides, chemicals) you take in, the more fat you need to store them. See how it works—more toxins, more fat, more toxins, more fat? This is your "toxic burden" and is one of the reasons why you are eating less, yet gaining weight and not feeling well.

When you combine your toxic burden with a lack of exercise,

consuming chemically laden "nonfoods," and ingesting loads of sugary delights, you will most likely end up with insulin resistance.

Insulin resistance leads to further cravings for sugary carbohydrates to generate energy for the body. Our poor diets started a vicious cycle beginning way back when we were young girls. These poor dietary habits are a setup requiring that more insulin be released in response to increased carbohydrate intake, which leads to *more* weight gain. More fat leads to more estrogens, which, in turn, leads to earlier breast development and onset of menstruation. Earlier onset of menstruation leads to more ovulatory cycles and a greater lifetime exposure to estrogens, and without adequate progesterone, which is, as we now understand, a dangerous condition called estrogen dominance, you could be in trouble healthwise. A greater lifetime exposure to estrogens without the protection of progesterone increases breast cancer risk.

Simultaneously, increased consumption of simple carbohydrates, coupled with insulin resistance, leads to polycystic ovary syndrome (PCOS) and a lack of ovulation during menstrual cycles; this state results in excess production of androgens and estrogens, and inadequate production of progesterone. Too much estrogen production and not enough progesterone can lead to estrogen dominance and increased breast cancer risk. When you add in the use of birth control pills (often prescribed for PCOS), insulin resistance can increase and exacerbate many of the problems above.

Our bodies require respect. You respect your body when you feed it right with real food and by exercising it regularly. When you are very young, you can get away with abusing your body; it's never good for you, but you can bounce back pretty quickly. As you enter your midthirties and early forties, you can't get away with it anymore.

Every choice you make from here on in will determine the

ease or *dis-ease* with which you enter perimenopause. Your body talks . . . all the time; it tells you what is working and what is not. Your body responds to everything you do for it, and everything you do to work against it. If you have gas and bloating, something you are eating is not agreeing with you. If you can't sleep, something is off in your body balance. If you are constipated, think back over your diet. What have you been eating? Ask yourself these questions on a regular basis.

The better you treat your body, the longer it will last and operate at peak. It's your body. You are in charge of how well it works . . . or doesn't.

## BE SMART ABOUT YOUR FOOD CHOICES

First of all, loss of hormones means you are transitioning into the next phase of your life. With perimenopause, every choice from this moment on will determine how well you age and the quality of your life. The good news . . . *you* are in charge of how well it goes. Educating yourself is the key. The abuse your body has withstood over the years from poor food choices, overconsumption of alcohol, and recreational stimulants will now take a toll. If you don't make smart food choices, you will wrinkle faster, your body will lose its shape, your health will degrade, and your sex drive will suffer.

So what are the smart choices to keep your body fit and in the best health and shape?

Smart food choices, supplementation, coupled with a natural hormonal regimen (which we'll explore later in the book) are the components to successfully navigating and enjoying perimenopause.

What do I mean by smart food and why does it matter?

Let's look at the benefits you get from just a single healthy meal.

Say you have finely chopped sautéed spinach or kale in olive oil with minced garlic, a medallion of wild caught salmon sautéed in olive oil and topped with crispy fried thin-sliced ginger and garlic, and a side of gluten-free pasta with roasted tomato sauce and sautéed pine nuts. (I know it's a lot of food, but I have a hearty appetite!) As soon as good (and might I add delicious) food gets put in your mouth and hits your saliva, your body begins working its magic and the process of digestion begins. Digestion extracts the nutrients from your food. Our bodies have learned how to benefit from the chemicals in food, discarding some and using others, as they see fit. Each of the extracted food chemicals interacts with other foods' chemicals and your own body's chemicals in very specific ways. It is a complex and magnificent process. Let's take a peek at the nutrients in just one of the foods in the preceding meal and why they're so good for you.

The spinach or kale alone is a cornucopia of various nutrients: calcium, iron, selenium, magnesium, phosphorus, potassium, vitamin K, vitamin A, vitamin E, vitamin C, $B_1$ (thiamin), $B_2$ (riboflavin), $B_3$ (niacin), $B_6$ (pyridoxine), fatty acids, amino acids, tryptophan, threonine, isoleucine, leucine, lysine, methionine, cysteine, phenylalanine, tyrosine, valine, arginine, histidine, alanine, aspartic acid, glutamic acid, glycine, proline, serine, and phytosterols! If we explore just one of these nutrients' benefits, phytosterols, you will see just how much real food really matters. Phytosterols are plant fat. They are the naturally occurring compounds within plants that act as a catalyst for certain plant cell functions. Ingesting phytosterols, in foods and in supplement form, may help you control your cholesterol levels. Phytosterols may also aid in joint health and in boosting your immune system.

The antioxidant effects of ginger, garlic, and turmeric are

tremendous. Antioxidants, in the simplest of terms, "eat" the free radicals (the bad guys) that bombard us each minute from living and from the toxins, chemicals, and pesticides that surround us. The more antioxidants you can take in, the better for your health.

Kale helps balance estrogen and wards off many forms of cancer, including breast, bowel, bladder, prostate, and lung cancers; it protects against heart disease and regulates blood pressure. The calcium in kale is easily absorbed by the body and protects against osteoporosis, arthritis, and bone loss. These are just the benefits in one dish; we haven't even touched on the rest of the foods in this meal.

It boggles the mind to see what nature has provided. You get a host of health benefits, including hormone-balancing ones, just from eating one serving of spinach or kale! Imagine what a regular diet of healthy foods can do for you? No need to imagine; next we are going to explore some key foods you'll want to stock up on.

## PERIMENOPAUSAL POWER FOODS

My idea of heaven is a great big baked potato and someone to share it with.

—Oprah Winfrey

It's important to know the jam-packed power of certain foods that will not only protect you from a myriad of health issues, but also will help you with hormone balance. Ideally, your food choices should be organic and pesticide free. Beef should be organic and grass-fed; fish should be wild not farm raised. It is difficult to get organic food at most restaurants, so when possible eat at home. When not, do your best.

## Almonds (raw, unsalted)

Almonds are a great source of protein, fiber, and minerals including:

Calcium and magnesium—Calcium keeps bones strong and promotes bone growth. Magnesium works in concert with calcium for bone growth and is a calming mineral needed by perimenopausal women. It is also good for assisting with constipation.

Iron— This mineral is necessary for transporting the active and usable form of thyroid, T3.

Potassium—Circulatory deficits happen with age and declining hormones; potassium ameliorates this by helping to support blood vessel health and reduce the risk of high blood pressure. A potassium-rich diet will prevent leg cramps and other muscle spasms. This is because of the role that potassium plays with muscle contraction and nerve impulses all over the body, including the heart.

Zinc—Research indicates that zinc helps balance female hormones, helps prevent PMS, and helps prevent acne.

Almonds are also high in vitamin E and unsaturated fats, keeping arteries supple. With the decline of minor hormones, cortisol goes high and is one of the main reasons women get (and die of) heart disease; almonds play a role in preventing atherosclerosis (hardening of the arteries).

## Apples

All types of apples contain quercetin, a powerful antioxidant that prevents the oxidation of LDL cholesterol, which in turn lowers the risk of damage to your arteries. An apple's pectin is effective in lowering levels of blood cholesterol.

### Avocado

This fruit may prevent breast cancer (*see* Brooke), as well as prostate cancer.

### Beans

Beans are loaded with complex carbohydrates, as well as calcium, iron, folic acid, B vitamins, zinc, potassium, and magnesium. They contain large amounts of soluble and insoluble fiber, which helps reduce cholesterol and normalize blood sugar.

### Beets

Beets contain high levels of carotenoids and flavonoids, which are known to protect artery walls as well as reduce the risk of heart disease and stroke. In addition, they contain iron and also boost bone health, due to their calcium content, thus reducing the risk of osteoporosis.

### Blueberries

Berries are a great source of antioxidants that keep your brain and heart healthier. Blueberries also contain pterostilbene, which is effective in reducing bad LDL cholesterol.

### Broccoli

This vegetable contains two powerful anticancer substances: sulforaphane and indole-3-carbinol. Sulforaphane destroys ingested carcinogenic compounds and kills *H. pylori* (*Helicobacter pylori*), a bacteria that causes stomach ulcers and increases the risk of gastric cancers. (If you eat in restaurants and consume non-organic chicken, it's likely at some point you will pick up *H. pylori*.) Indole-3-carbinol metabolizes estrogen, potentially protecting against estrogen dominance and breast cancer. It also has a good amount of potassium and beta-carotene.

### Cabbage

High in fiber, vitamin A, and minerals, cabbage stimulates the immune system, kills bacteria and viruses, inhibits growth of cancerous cells, protects against tumors, helps control estrogen levels and promotes balance, improves blood flow, and boosts sex drive. It speeds up the metabolism of estrogen toward a "good" metabolite and slows the production of a bad one, reducing the risk of breast cancer, and inhibits the growth of polyps in the colon; cabbage also protects against stomach ulcers.

### Eggs

Eggs are a good source of selenium, riboflavin, vitamin $B_{12}$, pantothenic acid, and vitamin D, and are rich in lutein and zeaxanthin (both offer protection for the eyes, which were not meant by nature to last beyond our childbearing years). Eggs are also a great source of choline, a neurotransmitter critical for brain health and a good source of natural progesterone.

### Flaxseed

This power food increases the number of ovulatory cycles in perimenopausal women and increases testosterone at the time of ovulation. Regular consumption of flaxseed improves the progesterone/estrogen ratio in postovulatory women and helps with PMS. Flaxseed is also an excellent source of essential omega-3 fatty acids. Freshly ground flaxseed releases more nutrients than whole flaxseed.

### Garlic

This yummy bulb is an excellent cancer fighter; it protects against cancers of the breast, colon, skin, prostate, stomach, and esophagus. Garlic stimulates the immune system by encouraging the growth of natural killer cells that directly attack cancer cells. Also, it has the ability to kill many of the antibiotic-resistant strains of MRSA (the hospital superbug).

### Meat

Lean meats (organic, of course, and grass-fed whenever possible) are an excellent source of protein. Meat also provides needed iron, $B_{12}$, and zinc. Bison meat is an often overlooked example of a healthier meat, because bison live on natural grass and spend very little time in feedlots or slaughterhouses. As such, they are not given drugs, chemicals, or hormones. Bison meat has a greater concentration of iron than any other meat, as well as some essential fatty acids. Of particular importance to women is its high iron content.

### Nuts

Nuts and seeds provide excellent nutritional value. They are especially good sources of essential fatty acids, gamma tocopherol vitamin E, protein, and minerals. They also provide valuable fiber components; important phytonutrients in nuts and seeds include protease inhibitors, ellagic acid, and other polyphenols.

## Olive Oil

Regular consumption of this omega-3-rich oil helps protect against heart attacks, because of its unique polyphenol and monounsaturated fatty-acid content. Polyphenols in extra virgin olive oil help keep cell membranes soft and pliable, allowing for oxygenation and hydration, the elements of life, to flow through the membranes easily and thus give energy and vitality.

## Oranges

Oranges contain high quantities of hesperetin, which protects against inflammation. Eating these regularly can lower cholesterol because of the fiber/pectin. They are a good source of potassium, which reduces blood pressure, as well as folic acid, which lowers levels of homocysteine (high levels of this substance in the body are not good for the heart).

## Pineapple

This is one of the top fifty foods with the highest antioxidant content. Antioxidants have been found to help protect cells from the damage of free radicals, which can break down muscles, increase aging effects, and as a result lead to cancers and other chronic diseases.

## Shellfish

These sea gifts are full of healthful vitamins and minerals. Oysters are a great source of vitamins A, $B_1$, $B_2$, $B_3$, and D and are also high in iron, calcium, magnesium, and other minerals. Many other shellfish are also excellent sources of iron and zinc, including mussels, clams, scallops, shrimp, prawns, and crab. Shellfish are one of the best dietary sources of zinc, a mineral necessary for keeping your immune system healthy and promoting the healing of wounds. The highest levels of zinc can be found in oysters.

### Sweet Potatoes

This power food is full of protein, fiber, artery-protecting beta-carotene, blood pressure–controlling potassium, and antioxidants.

### Tea

Black, green, and now white teas are hailed for their anti-oxidant properties. The polyphenols in green tea are powerful antioxidants and protect against free-radical damage, which is a major cause of arterial aging. Green tea may inhibit breast, digestive, and lung cancers as well.

### Tomatoes

Cooked tomatoes contain high levels of lycopene, a nutrient that reduces the risk of prostate, lung, and stomach cancers. Tomatoes contain potassium, vitamin C, and lycopene; each is essential to your immune system and to keep your skin healthy.

### Wild Salmon

This fish is an excellent source of omega-3 fatty acids. Eating omega-3 rich salmon regularly may help protect against heart disease, breast and other cancers, as well as provide relief to sufferers of certain autoimmune diseases, such as rheumatoid arthritis and asthma. Its omega-3s are great for mood and also protect the brain, and are essential for the membranes of every one of your 60 to 90 trillion or so cells in your body.

Do you see what eating the right foods can do for you? You can clearly see the difference between eating any of these power foods versus a fast-food hamburger from your local drive-in. Look at the nutrients your body misses by making the wrong food choices! How can you function at your prime without the right fuel?

## SUPPLEMENTING FOR OPTIMAL PERIMENOPAUSAL HEALTH

You shouldn't just rush out and grab every supplement we discuss in this book. That's not my aim, nor is it responsible. When creating a supplement regimen, team up with your doctor or a nutritionist and have him or her do blood work to tailor your intake to your individual needs.

### KEY NUTRIENTS FOR BALANCING HORMONES

Because I am not a doctor or nutritionist, I went to a trusted expert, Dr. Jonathan Wright, so he could share the most current information on which essential nutrients a perimenopausal woman may need. Dr. Wright, as past readers know, is the pioneer in this country of BHRT, and one of my most trusted sources of valuable information on female reproductive health.

**JW:** Back in the 1930s, it was found that if experimental animals were deprived of this one nutrient, called manganese, they simply couldn't reproduce anymore. They got everything else, but this one missing factor ceased reproduction. Fairly recently it was discovered that manganese in the hypothalamus stimulates luteinizing hormone-releasing hormone (LHRH), which then stimulates the pituitary to make luteinizing hormone.

**SS:** Why does this matter?

**JW:** The pituitary tells the ovaries to make progesterone. LH goes to the ovaries to instruct them to make progesterone.

**SS:** So if a woman is having trouble conceiving or with irregular periods, it could be that she is deficient in manganese?

**JW:** Yes, I would give these women manganese.

**SS:** That is pretty sophisticated detective work. I think of all the women going to fertility clinics, when it might be so simple.

Is there a connection between poor diet and premature perimenopause?

**JW:** Absolutely. Poor diet, environmental chemicals, and also the electromagnetic fields we all live in.

**SS:** What nutrients affect women's hormones?

**JW:** We talked a little about manganese, but there's more. Manganese stimulates progesterone in premenopausal and perimenopausal women. It stimulates luteinizing hormone-releasing hormone, which stimulates luteinizing hormone, which stimulates progesterone in women (and testosterone in men). Manganese is essential for strong bones, collagen formation, and proper brain function. Low levels of manganese can cause muscle contractions, vision and/or hearing loss, convulsions, rapid heart rate, and atherosclerosis. The daily recommendations are 10 milligrams of manganese. Great dietary sources of manganese are found in blueberries, various nuts, shellfish, egg yolks, pineapple, and avocados.

Then there's flaxseed: ground flaxseed in premenopausal women increases the number of ovulatory cycles, increases testosterone at the time of ovulation, and improves the progesterone/estrogen ratio in postovulatory women and helps PMS!

**SS:** It's also a good source of omega-3 and it helps to

keep you "regular." How much flaxseed should a woman eat daily?

**JW:** At least one ounce or 28 grams, that's about one rounded tablespoonful. You can either grind flaxseed yourself or buy it in sealed containers, already ground. Both are available at natural food stores, many supermarkets, the Tahoma Clinic Dispensary, and numerous online sources. If you buy it already ground, avoid large containers, so it won't have as much time to oxidize. Always make sure it's organic!

**SS:** What else do women need?

**JW:** Iodide/iodine. Iodine is necessary for the synthesis of thyroid hormones in both sexes. Iodine helps to prevent breast cancer by increasing estriol, a cancer-protective estrogen. Recent research shows that iodine combines with a specific lipid (a fat) in breast tissue. Researchers in Mexico, India, and Germany have proven that this combination (called an iodolactone) kills breast cancer cells. Shellfish are a great source of iodine; sea salt, seafood, seaweed, eggs, dairy products are all also rich with iodine.

**SS:** As a woman who once had breast cancer there is never a day I miss taking my iodine supplement.

**JW:** As you should; it's very important and especially important when women are estrogen dominant.

## SUPPLEMENTS TO CONSIDER

Supplements need to be determined by your deficiencies. This is done through blood work ordered by a qualified doctor or nutritionist. These experts can work out a supplementation regimen tailored just for you. Our soil and plants no longer have the sufficient nutrients so supplementation in today's world is crucial. Most perimenopausal women need to supplement iodine, calcium, magnesium, and omega-3 fish oil, which we have discussed. In addition, you may try the following:

## Acetyl-L-Carnitine (ALCAR)

This amino acid supplement is naturally produced by the liver and the kidneys, and helps the body turn fat into energy. For perimenopausal women this can be an important helper in combating the weight gain that accompanies this passage. When your muscles have enough ALCAR, they can easily burn fat or protein, and not just glucose, for energy. This sufficiency delays muscle fatigue, decreases lactic acid, and increases testosterone production (which boosts muscle and bone mass, as well as sex drive and mood).

But the benefits for the brain are the most exciting consequence of ALCAR. It is effective at passing the blood-brain barrier, which plays a role in producing acetylcholine, a neurotransmitter vital to the proper functioning of the brain and entire nervous system. With toxins attacking our brains in today's world, and brain cancers on the rise with younger and younger people, protecting your brain needs to be at the top of your list. When you are in your thirties and forties, brain damage seems to be something reserved for the very old. Again I say my peers—who are in various stages of brain damage, brain cancers, dementia, Alzheimer's, and find themselves sitting in nursing homes—likely never gave protecting their brains a thought. ALCAR is also essential for the mitochondria, which are the energy center of our cells. It allows for oxygen to reach your brain; if you get no oxygen to your brain, it stops functioning. Be smart. ALCAR is a small thing to take every day that may produce big results.

## Berry-Derived Anthocyandins

Anthocyandins are the red-blue pigments that give many plants their color. Berries are potent antioxidants. As mentioned earlier, antioxidants "eat" free radicals (toxins). Berries and the extracts derived from them, including resveratrol, promote heart health and protect cells from the mutation-inducing effects of toxic food preservatives. Since it's difficult to avoid food with preservatives, even for the health conscious, you see why this supplement is a necessary piece of your arsenal. You would have to eat a bushel basket of berries every day to get the dosage recommended by experts available in one daily supplement. Try Enhanced Berry Complete with RZD Acai from www.lef.org.

## Boron

The mineral boron raises estrogen and testosterone in pre-, peri-, and postmenopausal women. At the same time, it supports bone health in combination with calcium (women experience greater bone loss and do not absorb calcium as well as they age). Sufficient calcium intake from food can slow the rate of bone loss.

## Calcium

Women of childbearing age whose menstrual periods stop because they exercise heavily, eat too little, or both need sufficient calcium to cope with the resulting decreased calcium absorption, increased calcium losses in the urine, slowdown in the formation of new bone, and magnesium loss. Magnesium protects against brain damage and free-radical damage, and it provides protection against toxicity. Calcium should always be taken with magnesium.

## CoQ$_{10}$

Every cell in the body needs CoQ$_{10}$. It activates the mitochondria, the energy center of your cells. Without sufficient CoQ$_{10}$

you will lose vitality and energy and your aging will accelerate. Ubiquinol CoQ10 is the best form to take.

### Fish Oil

Fish oil may be the most important supplement you can take. The body requires a constant intake of essential fatty acids, or EFAs (they are called essential because they are indeed that important to life). Every cell is dependent on EFAs and they get burned up (oxidized) from everyday living. The more stress you are under, especially physical stress like exercise and dieting, the more aggressive you need to be about your EFAs and this great source of them, fish oil. Fish oil reduces inflammation as it circulates through the bloodstream. Since your blood is everywhere in your body, the anti-inflammatory effects of fish oil are far-reaching.

Fish oil, because of its omega-3 fatty acids specifically, has been used to treat depression and other mood disorders, as well as attention deficit disorder (ADD) and even bipolar issues. For perimenopausal women combating moodiness and depression, fish oil can go a long way to rectify these symptoms. It's hard to obtain consistent potencies of omega-3s by eating fish. So eating fish, sadly, is no longer the optimum source for EFAs due to mercury content, PCBs, and potential heavy metal contamination. Look for fish oil supplements that are 5-star IFOS (International Fish Oil Standards). If you are on daily aspirin or a blood thinner, please discuss first with your physician.

### N-Acetylcysteine (NAC)

Glutathione is the body's master antioxidant. NAC is rapidly metabolized in the body where it becomes a precursor to intercellular glutathione. Numerous studies have shown its power. It can improve heart function, blood sugar numbers in diabetics, and response to exercise. It is also excellent for detoxifying the intestinal tract, one of the premier residences for toxins, molds, and candida. Unfortunately, we stop manufacturing most glutathione around age thirty-five, so now we are left without this key defense against the greatest environmental assault of toxicity in the history of humankind. Our livers are groaning from trying to process toxins and poisons the body was never meant to handle. Just our morning ritual (showering, bathing, brushing teeth, using cosmetics) exposes the average person to over two hundred different toxins. In addition, we are exposed to over eighty thousand different toxins on a regular basis through sources such as these: the air we breathe, the water we drink, the fluoride (a known carcinogen) and chlorine (another known carcinogen) in our pools, the cleaning products we use to "sanitize" our homes, the air fresheners, the plastic water bottles emitting bisphenol As, dishwashing detergents, insect repellents, and other chemicals.

The need for protective supplements is great. If you want to achieve balance hormonally, you must take into account that the environment is working against you, not with you, so taking powerful antioxidant supplements will provide a lot of protection. Different antioxidants eat different free radicals, so taking a full course of antioxidants is advised. (That's why this list includes many different forms of antioxidant protection.)

## Vitamin D/D$_3$

Vitamin D/D$_3$ is a hormone. Let me explain what I mean by that. Early man (Paleolithic) walked naked in the sun taking in sufficient amounts of vitamin D the way nature had planned as the delivery system to keep the human body healthy. When sunlight strikes your skin, it passes through your liver and it is turned into 25-hydroxyvitamin D (this is what doctors measure to determine your vitamin D level). The kidneys then get into the action, supplying a small chemical adjustment that creates the active version of vitamin D. The active version of vitamin D is actually the hormone calcitriol, also known as vitamin D. Calcitriol is very powerful; it controls calcium and phosphorus absorption, bone metabolism, and neuromuscular function.

It is a hugely important supplement you should consider taking as soon as your doctor green-lights it. Vitamin D is essential to all the important systems in your body:

- Immune (you can't be healthy without a strong immune system)
- Endocrine (hormones)
- Cardiovascular (heart)
- Cognitive (the brain)

Vitamin D is associated with bone health because it helps your digestive system to absorb calcium and phosphorus, so a vitamin D deficiency is associated with osteoporosis and hip fractures. I realize you are only in perimenopause and you aren't worried about your bones, but think about this; neither were the older women of today whose bones are sometimes so weak they can't hold them up. Add to that hearts that are failing, brains that aren't firing, and bodies that are hormonally depleted. What we are talking about here is preventive medicine. Taking vitamin $D_3$ today could offset terrible health events later in your life. It's just smart to protect yourself.

Dozens of new studies have found that vitamin $D_3$ affects human health in much more profound ways than was ever imagined. It is now well established that the active form of vitamin $D_3$ acts as an effective regulator of cell growth and differentiation in a number of different cell types, including cancer cells. Vitamin $D_3$ protects us from the four most common cancers: breast, prostate, colon, and skin. If you are not taking a vitamin $D_3$ supplement or drinking a lot of milk fortified with vitamin $D_3$, or unless you can consciously lie naked in the sun for a minimum of twenty minutes daily (both sides), then you should seriously consider vitamin D replacement. Vitamin D is a hormone, so in turn it communicates with all the other hormones and is part of the hormonal song. As you are beginning to decline in other hormones at this passage, vitamin D is another of those that have gone missing and likely needs replacing.

## NEED A LIFT?—
## DIET, MOOD, AND DEPRESSION

Still not convinced it's worth giving up the junk and choosing better foods and nutrition for yourself? Understand that a poor diet leads to a body low or missing in minerals and needed nutrients, a body that just will not operate properly. With perimenopause already playing havoc with your body's balance and throwing everything off, it is vital to take diet and supplementation seriously. If not, serious conditions can result, including one of the most common complaints of this transition: depression. Understanding which nutrients you need to replace to combat depression will clear the way so you can have an easier time with perimenopause. So many women complain of depression during perimenopause. But did you know that not just hormonal decline can cause it? An imbalance of zinc and copper can also affect your mood states. If you are estrogen dominant, these two minerals may be significant factors, even though our bodies only need small amounts. The *balance* of these two minerals is key because they are cofactors for important enzymes that affect our mood.

Copper and zinc are involved in the function of the brain's cells. They are very important in the brain's regulation of mood, as well as its reaction to stress.

Researchers have noted that there's an association between high copper levels and low zinc levels during PMS. This copper and zinc imbalance can lead to depression. Excess estrogen raises the level of a copper-binding protein called ceruloplasmin in the bloodstream, which can also bind to copper and prevent it from getting into the brain cells where it is needed for proper enzyme function (*see* Clemente). The cellular levels of these minerals are controlled by the cell membrane. A healthy cell membrane allows just the right amounts of potassium, magnesium, copper, and zinc to be kept within the cell, while at the same time keeping the sodium out that would result in cell swelling. Progestins (pharmaceutical progesterone-like chemicals) impair this action of the cell membrane, whereas natural progesterone restores proper function of it.

You know now that a deficiency of zinc combined with excess copper can lead to severe mood disturbances and imbalances. If you are plagued by chronic depression, have your blood tested for these minerals. If you have imbalances of copper and zinc, balancing these levels will set things right in your brain and thus help you avoid the pitfall of so many women who become addicted to antidepressants. A qualified doctor will understand the need for blood testing to look for any deficiencies in your body. If you want your body to operate at max, it requires constant detective work to analyze what needs replacing.

Whenever you can get these missing minerals and vitamins from food it is always best. Foods that contain high levels of zinc include shellfish, as stated earlier, and the lean muscle tissues, or tenderloin, of beef, deer, or lamb. Every 4 ounces of beef tenderloin contains about 5 mg of zinc. Tenderloin can be easily added to meals and snacks. Zinc can also be found in pumpkin and sesame seeds, containing 2.5 mg and 2.8 mg of zinc per $^1/_4$ cup, respectively. Sesame seeds can easily be added to yogurt or baked goods. Pumpkin seeds can be purchased from any health food store or harvested from a pumpkin and toasted.

Avoid raw, unprocessed soy products as they contain high levels of phytates that directly block the absorption of zinc. Fermented soy products, soy protein isolate, and soy isoflavones do not contain high levels of phytates. It's important to look for non-GMO soy products.

# CHAPTER 6

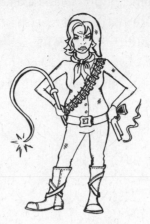

# GET MOVING—AND OTHER LIFESTYLE
# SHIFTS TO CONSIDER

If you rest, you rust.

—Helen Hayes

If you want to feel better and prime your body to be its healthiest, there are two lifestyle shifts that are imperative: You have to move. And you have to sleep. You can't be truly healthy without both.

If you had a brand-new car, but you never drove it and it just sat in your garage, when you finally did decide to take it out for a spin, it would sputter and choke. It wouldn't work as well. Cars need to be driven; they need to move to keep their parts lubricated and in top form. Your body works the same way; we were meant to move. Early man hunted and gathered; being fit was essential for survival. I'm pretty sure there were no fat people in Paleolithic times; they didn't have processed foods and gluten orgies. Their lives were about surviving; they ate only what they needed (or could find), and exercise was just a normal part of going about their lives. They didn't fear some of the things we commonly do; instead they were dodging large animals who considered them prey. So it was imperative they be in top form or risk being eaten.

Perimenopause brings with it a host of built-in excuses for not exercising:

It won't matter, I'm fat anyway.

I didn't sleep last night, and I'm just too tired.

I'm in a bad mood and nothing will help it.

I don't have time.

I'm too busy.

I'm too . . . everything.

The biggest excuse (and rightfully so) is that you are in peri-menopause. This life passage zaps your energy and affects your mood. Hormones are the rulers of the body and right now you don't have enough or you have none. Hormones are called "the juice of youth" because they give you all the great feelings you have been used to having all your life . . . until now. Without them you aren't the same person. Don't worry and don't be so hard on yourself. You are going to get them back and then some.

Nothing will help you get all your hormones working better than exercise. When you add hormone replacement to the mix, you will be amazed that your body, mood, life quality, and sex drive will be back better than ever.

There will always be excuses, reasons, and obstacles in our way on any given day. But it's a fact: exercise just makes the body work better. Exercise oxygenates the body and tells the brain that we are alive. The more you exercise, the more energy you have to *want* to exercise.

I'm basically lazy . . . I love to lie in bed in the morning and drink my cup of coffee, watch the morning news, hang out with Alan, play around with my cats, and noodle on my iPad. I have to force myself to be disciplined. I made a commitment to myself some years ago that I would exercise every weekday morning. It's not formal. Sometimes I throw in a mountain hike. My bedroom faces the mountains, and as I lie in bed early mornings there are days the beautiful mountains beckon me. I put on my hiking shoes and the moment I am on a trail I feel like I am in church, looking at all the wondrous things of nature along the way.

On weekends, I do lie around. I hang out in bed with Alan until as late as eleven o'clock, and I find that to be very enriching for both us. To have two days a week where we don't leap out of bed to begin "activities" is both a treat and a luxury. It allows us to recharge.

At my age *not* exercising is a setup for poor health and a flabby-looking body. Wait until you hit sixty-six; the game really changes. But I do believe all the exercise I did for twenty-five years as a Vegas headliner prepped my body for this present passage of my life when everything about staying fit and healthy is harder. In other words, the exercise you do today will have a big payoff down the road.

I believe I am aging well. I feel good, and I like the way I look. It didn't happen by accident. I put work into this project and have found for myself exercises that I enjoy. Sitting in front of your computer all day leaves you short on energy and vitality, but the reality is that sitting is our new way of life. As humans in the modern world we aren't working in the fields; instead, we sit and stare at our computer screens, sometimes for hours and then get up at the end of the day feeling stiff. Here is where yoga is your friend. Many of us mistakenly feel that if we don't do a workout that lasts hours, it's worthless. So we do nothing instead.

It's more important that you do a little exercise regularly than that you try to break any endurance records. There's no failing grade; the only way you fail is by doing nothing at all. Short exercise sessions are just as beneficial as long ones. Why not do several five-minute sessions throughout the day? You can walk around the block. Do wall pushups. Stand up for phone calls. Whatever works for you.

I have a glider, an EZGym, a thigh trainer, a Thigh-master (had to get that one in here), free weights, and my yoga mats, yoga balls, and yoga straps. I'm never bored regardless of what I choose to do that day. I enjoy all my forms of exercise. I get lost in thought on the glider, I get spiritually inspired on a hike, and I am intensely aware of every breath, every muscle, every challenge in yoga. Yoga asks that you put your thoughts or brain "noise" aside for an hour and just focus on doing each move, using your breath as deeply as you can. I usually do yoga three times a week. It makes my body toned, stretched, and lengthened, and yoga helps sculpt a beautiful feminine body. Yoga keeps your body long and lithe and your butt high and firm. (Believe me, nothing ages a woman more than having a flat shapeless butt!) At the end of my yoga practice, I lie on the mat and usually meditate for five minutes. It's restful and calming.

Perimenopause inherently brings anxiety, so exercise is your ticket to staying calm. Also, with constipation being something I hear about from my readers on a regular basis at this age, there is no better way to get things "moving" than to exercise and drink a lot of water.

Most nights before I go to bed I do three or four rounds of free weights. It only takes me five minutes and I don't use particularly heavy weights: 5 pounds for flys, 10 pounds for biceps curls, 5 pounds for lunges. Most people think I am a fitness fanatic, but as you can see, that is not true. I find the easiest way possible to get movement in each day. I always search for something I find pleasurable. All in all I probably put in a total of forty minutes of exercise a day but I do it in spurts so it doesn't feel regimented. I enjoy my short spurts. I don't know about you, but I do not have the time to put on a little outfit, drive to the local gym, exercise for an hour or so, shower, and then drive home. That's half a day right there! I don't have a half a day to give to exercise. So I grab it in pieces all throughout the day and I enjoy it much more.

## DO YOU HAVE A FEW HOURS TO EXERCISE . . . EACH WEEK?

A study out of King's College in London found that people who exercised vigorously three hours a week were biologically nine years younger than those who exercised fewer than fifteen minutes a week. Most people feel they have to join a gym and spend endless hours a week. But 3 hours out of 168 in a week is absolutely doable, especially when broken up!

## STAND UP OR STIFFEN UP

Our sedentary lifestyles are doing us in. Our hips are widening, our stomachs are getting flabby, our arms are losing tone. Our necks get tight and our backs get weary from jobs that don't make us move. If you have stairs in your home, you are lucky, as they force you to do at least something!

It's no joke, being sedentary will cause you to eventually stiffen up, just like it would if you never drove your car; it would sputter and groan when you finally chose to drive it. When you don't move your lymphatic system, it doesn't work properly. The lymph glands are responsible for moving debris (toxins) out of the body and also to move hormones around! The lymph is your transport system. Nature did not provide a "pump" for the lymph system as it has for the heart and the circulatory system. Nature presumed that walking, hunting, and gathering would keep the lymph flow going.

You can see what being sedentary does to your hormonal flow. This should be motivation to get moving. By not moving, your moods are affected, your libido is affected, your hormones are affected, and your body won't look as good. Exercise is like saving for retirement . . . the more you consistently do something physical, anything, the better you will look, the more energy you will have, and the longer you will most likely live! Consistent exercise makes your figure look better and better, your posture improves, and your mood is improved. There's even research documenting that exercise can be as, if not more, effective for treating depression than prescription antidepressants . . . and it's certainly a lot healthier for you.

Another benefit of exercise is that your body's metabolism continues to operate at a faster rate long after the actual exercise. The combined effect of naturally released HGH (human growth hormone) and the increased need to repair and recover from high-intensity workouts lead to incredible fat burning. You become faster, leaner, stronger, and fitter as a result of the recovery or downtime, not the actual exercise itself.

## DON'T FEEL LIKE EXERCISING?
## IT MIGHT BE YOUR HORMONES

Hormones play a huge role in how you feel and your willingness or desire to exercise. When balanced, you're energized and ready to go. But if not, it's easy to let it slide, and then unbalanced hormones begin a cascade where because you don't exercise you have decreased muscle mass, then these things happen:

- Decreased muscle mass leads to a diminished ability to burn fat, resulting in weight gain.
- Decreased production in HGH leads to loss of lean muscle and increased body fat.
- Estrogen levels drop. Since estrogen is required for optimal thyroid function, when estrogen levels drop, your thyroid function decreases and weight gain can result (*see* Menna).

It's interesting that declining hormones seem to have a goal and that is to keep us fat. The only thing I can think of is nature in its wisdom is trying to "pad us up" so that our now becoming-brittle bones will have some padding to protect us if we fall. I guess that's nice?

Don't let that happen. Take exercise seriously.

## BEFORE YOU START

Before you start a new exercise regimen, first assess any health restrictions with your doctor. If you haven't exercised in forever, a basic physical that measures your organ function and explores any chronic ailment or lingering pains is a good idea. You don't want to invite injury by overdoing it with a body part that has been underused or has an underlying weakness.

Start slowly. Get up to a decent level of fitness before you push really hard. This is especially true with resistance training. I watched this happen with my husband who hadn't used weights for some time and went back to it with the full-strength weights he had worked with previously. Full out, he did biceps curls and overhead lifts until a sharp pain in his shoulder stopped him. He had shoulder problems for months after that, and even now a year later he still has to baby that shoulder. Take a lesson from him: overdoing it before you are ready will work against you.

## WHAT'S THAT MUSCLE?

Muscle fibers come in three different types: slow-burning, fast-burning, and strength-endurance. Slow-burning muscle fibers burn fat and oxygen and give us our energy for our activities throughout the day. Recreational and varied sports use the slow-burning muscles for weekend athletics like baseball, volleyball, and swimming. Knowing that there are these three types of focus for muscles has given my workout program an objective. I have chosen types of exercise to stimulate all three forms.

Fast-burning muscle fibers burn off sugar and store short-term energy sources such as creatine, but they burn almost no fat. They kick in when you need explosive, fast, or very powerful, rapid reactions. Strength-endurance fibers use both sugar and fat for fuel. These fibers allow us to intensify the exercise effort to somewhere between comfortable and maximum, and sustain it for a while. They are best worked through cardio and aerobic training.

This is important so you can balance your workouts and challenge all three muscle fibers to grow. In my case, walking and yoga is where I get my slow burning. Weights, swimming, and hiking are my fast *and* slow burning, and the glider is where I use the last five minutes to do my full-out strength endurance. By that time I can't wait to go full out.

If your workout is focused on slow-burning muscles, they are the only ones that benefit. If your workout is focused only on fast-burning fibers, your body responds by trying to get both the slow-burning and the strength-endurance muscles to do more of the work. Your body hates the maximum-intensity exercises because it requires extra energy, so it looks for as much support as possible from the other fibers. Most of us don't usually engage in the kind of intensity that shocks our bodies into extreme energy output; as a result we develop a slow-burning crisis. (That's when you walk up the hill and feel out of breath, or find using the stairs is too much effort.) Over the years most of us lose much of our fast-burning and explosive muscle fibers. This makes moving quickly too much of an effort, even though we may be able to jog for hours at a time at a moderate pace. The good news is even if you haven't been exercising and these muscles have become dormant, by exercising (and starting slowly) you can reengage and reinvigorate them. Full-out endurance exercises are saved for the end of your workout, allowing you to get out of breath, really working the heart and the muscle fibers. Maybe you are on the Stairmaster, or the walking machine at the gym if that is what you choose. They all have a maximum speed. Work up to it as best you can, slowly building your endurance. This is maxing your muscle potential. The more of this you do, the more you will be able to do.

## WHAT EXERCISES TO DO

Working these muscles can be accomplished beautifully with the following exercises.

### Yoga

Any kind will benefit you. You can go to a class, buy a DVD or video, have a private instructor, or purchase a yoga mat and do the daily stretches and routines at home. Yoga will give you a slow-burning workout, while gently stretching and lengthening each of your muscle sets.

## Resistance Training

The resistance in resistance training comes from pitting the muscles against a force, usually a weight such as a dumbbell or even the weight of your own body. Weight training is something you should do all the way to and through your nineties and longer. Lifting weights encourages bone growth by pulling the muscles against the bone. Bones have osteoclasts and osteoblasts, which are also stimulated by sufficient estrogen, progesterone, and testosterone. As we discussed earlier, testosterone is an anabolic steroid that stimulates the growth of bone and muscle.

Don't worry about the amount of weight; as I mentioned, I use 5-pound weights for flys. But once a weight poundage gets "easy," then you know it's time to go up a pound or two. You will never regret doing weightlifting. Your beautiful arms, butt, and legs will thank you over and over. (So will your partner.) This is the exercise that will stimulate your fast-burning muscle fibers.

## Cardio

Endurance is required if you are going to do cardio. These exercises make you winded, and that is the objective: to pump up the heart and get it pounding. This year I started doing dance classes with a DVD that I pop into my computer. I featured exercise dancers on my Lifetime talk show and I couldn't help but notice that they were having so much fun. They danced like it wasn't even exercise. It inspired me, so now I'm dancing several times a week and loving it. It feels effortless, because it's fun. It oxygenates my body, making me feel really alive. Aging people often lose vitality because of a lack of oxygenation due to low cardio output. Keeping your heart pumping regularly will change that.

With a dance exercise DVD, you start slowly, and build over time to full out. Recently, my producers planned a flash mob at

Universal Studios in Hollywood, and suddenly about five hundred people started dancing full out to "Crazy Love." It only lasted two minutes, but I was winded, my heart was beating wildly, and I was laughing hysterically because it was so much fun. Each time I do dance exercises I get better and faster and less winded with less internal burning. This allows me to know I am building my cardio, which helps with every facet of health in my body: the lymph system is activated, which is crucial for health.

Women die of heart disease; it is our biggest killer. Anything you can do to keep your heart muscles in shape will work in your favor. It's not too early; starting now gives you a huge head start. Extreme cardio exercises the heart muscle, giving you more endurance. Your skin also benefits, and your hormones get activated to operate at prime. Warm up before you start regardless of your fitness level.

For more cardio: dancing, walking, running, gliding, Stairmaster, Zumba, running up and down stairs at work or at home. Keep increasing your cardio until you feel your chest pounding. Try vigorous swimming or treading water until you can't anymore or hiking so you can enjoy the outdoors. Here is where you get in your strength endurance and aerobics. Near the end of your workout see what your body can do. Leave yourself breathless. Start with one minute and work up.

When you see old people shuffling across the street, with their heads down, out of breath, aching bones and joints, moving slowly, wearing too many clothes because they are cold even on the hottest days, it's because their circulation is shot from a lack of oxygen. It is clear they gave up exercising and oxygenating their bodies long ago. By exercising throughout your life your bones will stay stronger, your energy will last, and your brain will work better. All pretty important stuff. My visual of myself at one hundred is this energetic old lady who's not "old."

## EATING FOR ENERGY AND REPAIR

The process of recovery and repair also needs nutritional help: lots of protein, more than what is contained in the carbohydrate-rich diet that most of us consume, and enough vitamins and minerals to help our cells be efficient at repair. I can't put enough emphasis on the food you feed your body. Good-quality protein after a workout actually continues the benefits of your exercise. Grass-fed beef, organic chicken, wild-caught fish, and organic eggs are great sources of proteins. After a strenuous workout, don't neglect to eat protein. And don't forget your veggies. Organic green leafy vegetables will keep your skin looking fresh and glowing, and your glands and organs will respond by working at optimum.

## SLEEP—MISS IT?

There is another factor in perimenopause that I hear about from my readers over and over—being unable to sleep. It's a cruel and harsh wake-up call that something is amiss. Sleep and declining hormones and an inability to have the energy to exercise are all intertwined. At first you think it's because you have so many to-do lists in your head, but when it becomes chronic you know something about your life has changed. IT'S YOUR HORMONES!

Remember when you used to go to bed and it never entered your mind that you wouldn't go to sleep? Lack of sleep degrades our health, zaps our energy, leaves us susceptible to disease, and keeps us from feeling happy or "right." Sleep is the game changer. Those who don't or can't sleep, left unchecked and addressed, unfortunately go down first. The body *requires* sleep.

Those who say they only need five hours or less nightly are fooling themselves.

Some women can't *get* to sleep and others can't *stay* asleep. Some women find they wake up off and on all night long. Either of these scenarios is miserable. Besides deteriorating your health it deteriorates your looks. Nothing will accelerate aging faster than lack of sleep.

Women often speak to me of the anxiety of bedtime, hoping they will sleep and then the disappointment of not being able to make it happen. Waking up in the middle of the night is a classic pattern of the hormone imbalance that rears its ugly head in perimenopause. This insomnia is not caused by anxiety or a racing mind. Instead this is a low estrogen/high cortisol event. You feel tired and exhausted but simultaneously incredibly awake and alert. Many women decide it's better to get up and work rather than lie there in the dark tossing and turning. High cortisol is the culprit. Remember that high cortisol makes sleep impossible. You want your cortisol to come down at night so you can go to sleep.

Here are some things you can do to set things right and sleep through the night.

### Sleep in the Dark— Leave Your Handheld in the Living Room

Cortisol reacts to light. Because we have our lights on till the wee hours, cortisol doesn't have a chance to go down naturally, and then when your minor hormones are declining as in perimenopause, the cortisol stays high all the time.

In one study, researchers put test subjects in a completely darkened room except for a pin light on the backs of their knees. When the skin "read" the light on the back of the knees, the subjects' cortisol went up. So leave your phone and your electronics out of the bedroom.

### Prepare to Sleep

At dusk, turn down the lights, and create an air of calmness in your home. Light candles. It's romantic, but even better, your cortisol "recognizes" that low lights mean it's time to rest. Just with this one change, you can begin to lower your cortisol.

### Don't Drink Before Bed

Alcohol is not good for sleep. Choose your nights to drink wisely. Alcohol reduces the amount of time you spend dreaming. The same goes for benzodiazepines. More on that next.

### Do Not Take Sleeping Pills

Benzodiazepines are a class of drugs that produce central nervous system (CNS) depression and that are most commonly used to treat insomnia and anxiety. There is the potential for dependence on and abuse of benzodiazepines, particularly by individuals with a history of multisubstance abuse. Alprazolam (Xanax), lorazepam (Ativan), clonazepam (Klonopin), diazepam (Valium), and temazepam (Restoril) are the five most prescribed, as well as the most frequently sold, benzodiazepines in the illicit drug market.

So many doctors haphazardly prescribe sleeping pills or benzodiazepines. These were originally only meant to be taken for a short period of time, but many people take them for months on end. When people take drug medications for months at a time, they are likely to become resistant to them and require higher doses to relieve their insomnia. Eventually they may become dependent on them. If they try to withdraw, they are likely to experience rebound anxiety, a reaction typified by anxiety, fatigue, insomnia, and irritability. The temptation to go back on the pills can be strong.

These drugs do not promote sleep, but rather a suspended bodily state. You are not getting the real hormone healing benefits of sleep on sleep medication. A deficiency of REM sleep can cause memory problems and varying degrees of physical and psychic disturbances. In fact, research shows that animals kept from dreaming several weeks in a row die prematurely. Become dependent on drugs and the chemical molecules have a cumulative negative effect on your health. Sleep the natural way and live long and healthy.

### Take an Epsom Bath

Now fill the bathtub with very warm water and put in Epsom salts. Epsom is mostly magnesium, and magnesium calms the body and also makes you regular so it's a win/win. Soak for twenty minutes to get the best effect of the salts.

### Consider GABA and Melatonin

Consider two chewable GABA tablets (available at health food stores). GABA, or gamma amino butyric acid, helps calm and relax us and is essential for the proper function of the brain and central nervous system. If you find you are up at night with your brain spinning from one thing to the next, try GABA to calm any "noise" in your brain.

Melatonin is the hormone of sleep. Melatonin has none of the negative side effects associated with traditional sleep medications. It is secreted from the pineal gland, which is located in the brain (very small amounts of melatonin are also produced in the retina and GI tract). The main function of the pineal gland is to help govern biological rhythms, such as the sleep-wake cycle. Researchers see this gland as important in coordinating and controlling our other hormone-release and immune responses. The pineal gland communicates with these other systems through the messenger melatonin. The pineal gland "knows" how old we are and when we are past our prime. It responds by producing lower levels of melatonin, which signals our other systems to break down and cause us to age. (Again, it's nature's way of trying to get rid of us and make room for the young reproductive ones.) If we can keep melatonin raised to optimal levels, we can once again trick our bodies into believing that we are still young. With optimal levels of melatonin, we can continue to produce high levels of sex hormones and keep our bodies operating with a well-functioning immune system to fight off disease. Chronologically we may be older, but biologically we will be younger.

Melatonin is synthesized from an amino acid called tryptophan, which in turn is converted into the brain chemical serotonin. Ultimately, serotonin is turned into melatonin. See how all hormones speak to one another? With adequate amounts of melatonin, you sleep soundly and deeply and you dream and wake up rested in the morning.

Consider a time-release melatonin capsule (my website offers a supplement called Sleep Renew). If you still need additional help, buy LifeWave nanotechnology sleep patches called Silent Night (there is a link to these on my website as well). These are nondrug patches that shrink the time it takes for the natural melatonin to pour.

## Go to Bed at Nine

As night falls, melatonin release induces sleep. Dawn shuts it
off, waking us up in the morning. As you now know, melatonin
is produced naturally in the body. Aging, work, travel, and stress
can cause changes in sleep patterns and are likely to have adverse
effects on melatonin secretion. If you go to bed three hours before
midnight, you can achieve optimal release of melatonin. These
three hours of melatonin production reset prolactin production.
Prolactin is the hormone nursing mothers make; it is secreted by
the pituitary gland and stimulates lactation (milk production). It
also has many other functions, including essential roles in the
maintenance of the immune system. Abnormally high prolactin
can delay puberty, interfere with ovulation in women, decrease libido in men, and decrease fertility. Elevated prolactin (hyperpro-
lactinemia) may be due to a benign tumor in the pituitary gland
called a prolactinoma. Three hours of melatonin production is always followed by six hours of prolactin production at night to rev
up the defensive arm of your immune system. If you don't go to
bed three hours before midnight, you only provoke one and a half
hours of prolactin production, resulting in possibly suppressing
your immune system.

You might be thinking, *How can I go to bed at nine p.m.? I
have so much to do. Plus, I'm not tired yet.* I hear this all the time. I
remember when I had to make this change. It's interesting how a
cancer diagnosis becomes a strange gift. When I was diagnosed,
I had to do some deep soul searching. What had I done in my
diet and lifestyle habits that allowed me to play host to this large
tumor in my breast? As I honestly assessed my habits I was ap-
palled. I had not taken diet seriously at that time. And I did not
take sleep seriously. Sleep was a nuisance that took me away from
the things I had to do. Of the books I've written, half were writ-

ten (in longhand) when the house went to sleep. If my husband got into bed to watch TV and fell asleep at nine o'clock, that's when I would go to my office to write. It was quiet, no phone calls, no distractions, and kids were asleep or doing schoolwork. I would stay up routinely until 3:00 a.m., then fall into bed and sleep until seven.

The body requires seven to eight hours nightly to be healthy, so imagine what I was doing to myself by only sleeping on average four hours nightly. My immune system was shot. Simultaneously, I was doing two different TV series plus traveling on weekends to do my "nightclub" act. Yes, in many ways this was a delicious and amazing experience; but it was also one that kept me and my endorphins revved up till all hours of the morning. I was young I thought. I was in my early forties. I was invincible. But then . . .

## YOU HAVE CANCER!

Those are words you never want to hear, but sadly, one out of three of you reading this will hear those words. (According to the American Cancer Society, a woman's lifetime risk of developing any cancer is 1 in 3, and 1 in 8 for breast cancer.) When I was diagnosed, I decided to change my life. I was going to eat as though my life depended on it. I was going to force myself to sleep eight hours nightly. I was going to balance my hormones with bio-identicals. I was not going to take either pharmaceutical or over-the-counter drugs, so my devotion to the first two promises was essential to my life and being able to survive and live.

Now, I look forward to taking care of myself. I look forward to getting into bed each night. I have shifted my thinking. I slip into those sheets every night, all clean and smelling good, and feel grateful that I have this chance at restoring and resting my body, the machine that houses *who I am!* The best thing I ever did for myself was relearn to sleep eight hours a night.

I turned my health and life around. So can you, even without such a dire diagnosis. If you follow the above advice, you should be able to get into bed and fall into a deep and restful sleep. The combination of these things will eventually retrain your body to sleep. Soon you will be looking forward to going to bed. I rarely wake up in the middle of the night now, and it has improved my looks, mood, and weight.

## MOST IMPORTANT, LIVE YOUR LIFE

Think of me like an older sister or aunt, one who is going to always talk straight to you.

Let me tell you what I know in its simplest form:

This transition will all pass once you get balanced. All will then be right.

Many women in hormonal decline become so unhappy during this passage that they end up destroying what they have worked for all their lives. Don't let that be you. Here's some advice, so you don't go there.

### Make Time for Romance

Not sex per se, but intimate time with your partner. Set the table beautifully, put the kids to bed, and make time for your loved one. Include candlelight, a meal made with love, and dessert. How about enjoying a yummy panna cotta with fresh raspberry sauce? Indulge. You spend so much of your life denying. Have some fun. If you are real busy, and the thought of cooking horrifies you, your slow cooker is your friend. Find recipes that you love (there are so many online) and just put ingredients in the pot early in the morning, turn to low, and eight hours later you have a meal that will elicit raves.

### Make Time to Truly Live, Not Just Rush

Take time to notice the beautiful flowers, the blooming of the trees. Take walks in the park. Call your parents and tell them you love them. Rekindle old friendships.

### Get Out of Your Head

I know it's not always the kindest place to be, but you have the power within you to push away the blues and the anger. You can make your life beautiful. Trust that your life is about to get back on track.

### Get Help If You Need It

If you truly don't think you can hold it together at this time, don't go it alone. Find a good therapist who will help you unravel the layers of your life to allow you to see what you have and who you are more clearly. I have been going to therapy off and on since I was a teen. There's no shame in taking care of yourself. Don't buy into that false belief. Biochemically, your hormones are pushing you, and replacement will get you out. But emotionally you need to nurture yourself to bring you all the way home. Tell yourself over and over until you know it, until you truly believe it: you are a wonderful and worthwhile person. You just happen to be a good person who has been going through a difficult time. You're not alone, and it's not your fault.

## Practice Gratitude

I'll say it again. We are composed of approximately sixty to ninety trillion cells. Every cell communicates with one another. Each morning (and I never miss doing this) I isolate just "one" of those cells and I tell 'it' how grateful I am for my life. I express how grateful I am for the love of my husband, my family, my work, my good health, and that I live in freedom in this great country. I then envision that one cell telling *all* the other cells in the body: "We're so happy; we are grateful; we are healthy. We have love." All cells communicate with one another so they all "hear" this daily message. It sounds simple, and maybe even a little unusual, but it is the most gratifying exercise of my day. It changes any bad mood, anxiety, panic, or stress I might be feeling. It only takes a few minutes. All you have to do is close your eyes, and do it. Stand in the morning light if you can as you do, for an added boost. Afterward, I am left for the day feeling happy and upbeat. Try it. It's magical.

> We choose our lives. Choose happiness and balance.
> Then go live your happy life!

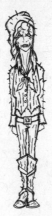

# CHAPTER 7

# I'M AFRAID TO TAKE HORMONES— WHAT THE RESEARCH REALLY SAYS ABOUT SYNTHETIC VERSUS BIOIDENTICAL HORMONES

*The standard policy of doctors is to be down on what they are not up on.*

—Dr. Garry Gordon, MD, DO

There is so much misinformation put out about hormones. One day headlines in the newspapers praise synthetic hormone replacement therapy (HRT). They proclaim the effectiveness of synthetic HRT in treating heart disease, osteoporosis, and Alzheimer's. The next day headlines are screaming that synthetic HRT may not benefit the above conditions and in fact will give you cancer!

The truth is, all hormones are not equal; also, not all hormones are used effectively by doctors to address the many diseases and conditions people suffer from. Most doctors are not skilled in hormone replacement and fewer still specialize in the use of bio-identical hormones to address the many diseases we face. (This is why the ForeverHealth.com network was created so women could have a site to find a qualified, vetted doctor who specializes in BHRT in an area nearest to them.)

First, let's clear up the confusion regarding synthetic hormones and bioidentical hormones.

## HOW THE USE OF SYNTHETIC HORMONES BEGAN

The first synthetic hormone, called DES (diethylstilbestrol), was invented in 1938. This pill was a carcinogenic monster of a hormone approved by the FDA in 1941 and given to millions of women from 1940 until it was banned in 1975, when it was proven to cause cervical cancer. From about 1940 to 1970, DES was given to pregnant women in the mistaken belief that it would reduce the risk of pregnancy complications and losses. In 1971, DES was shown to cause a rare vaginal tumor in girls and women who had been exposed to this drug in utero. The FDA subsequently withdrew DES from use in pregnant women. Follow-up studies have indicated DES also has the potential to cause a variety of significant adverse medical complications during the lifetimes of those exposed.

Next, the drug industry invented Premarin, a horse estrogen isolated from the urine of pregnant horses. Its name was derived from "pre" (for pregnant) "mare" (horse). The problem is a horse has at least ten different estrogens, most of which are not common to the human female. But that's just a minor detail. At least that's how Pharma seemed to see it and handle it.

Premarin was approved by the FDA in 1942 and became available to women that year. Premarin has caused an estimated fifteen thousand cases of endometrial cancer during the five-year period between 1971 and 1975 alone. This represents a huge epidemic of serious disease caused as a side effect of a prescription drug (*see* Jick). You'd think this would put an end to this nasty drug but no. Pharmaceutical companies brought us Prempro as a fix. This time the "prem" was for Premarin and the "pro" for progestin.

The drug industry's researchers decided that adding to the mix a "fake" progesterone, a synthetic *progestin*, medroxyprogesterone acetate, would rehabilitate Premarin. So instead of a drug that contained only horse estrogen, we now had access to another fake hormone. This was meant to make it more effective and safer, and this combo was meant to prevent endometrial cancer. Again, the FDA approved Prempro, and it was handed out to millions of women.

But uh-oh! Unsurprisingly, there were problems again. Four large-scale studies showed an increase in breast cancer and heart disease from taking this combo pill. Follow-up data from The Breast Cancer Detection Demonstration Project, published in the *Journal of the American Medical Association* in 2000, showed an eightfold increase in breast cancer for estrogen-progestin users (*see* Schairer)! That was the tip of the iceberg; other studies cited the following:

- The Swedish Record Review in 1996 showed a 40 percent increase in liver and colon cancer with this drug (*see* Persson).
- The Million Women Study, published in *The Lancet* in 2003, showed a 65 percent increase in breast cancer for estrogen-progestin combination users compared to estrogen alone users (*see* Beral).
- The final death blow to this drug should have come when the famous Women's Health Initiative study came out in

2002 (*see* Rossouw). It did put the use of synthetics in jeopardy, too. The study determined that those taking synthetic estrogen and progestin had an increased risk of heart disease and increased breast cancer. *The study was stopped because the researchers believed these health risks outweighed the drugs' benefits.*

Prior to the Women's Health Initiative (WHI), it was believed by many in the medical establishment that these hormones would decrease incidences of breast cancer, stroke, pulmonary embolism, colorectal cancer, endometrial cancer, hip fracture, and death due to any cause.

But the results and the actual outcome were astonishing! Researchers saw a

- 29 percent increase in coronary heart disease
- 41 percent increase in strokes
- 22 percent increase in cardiovascular disease
- 200 percent increase in lung and blood clots
- 26 percent increase in breast cancer

Now what could a woman do?

The findings of the WHI were not news to some in the medical community. In fact, many other studies (including some listed above) had already suggested the negative influences synthetic hormones (commonly called HRT for hormone replacement therapy) had on cardiovascular disease, strokes, blood clots, and cancer.

The information exposed by this study made international headlines. It made such an impact that it had physicians and patients questioning the safety and efficacy of these medications and rushing to get off them.

No wonder women decided to throw away their hormones!

Women felt betrayed, like we drank the Kool-Aid. We trusted, because after all, Premarin and Prempro had become such a prominent treatment for menopause and osteoporosis in our society. And to make matters worse, many unsuspecting doctors freely gave these drugs to us.

After WHI, women who had taken the synthetic hormones did something unprecedented; realizing that the FDA was not protecting them, they hired lawyers. Over thirteen thousand women have filed cases in court claiming synthetic hormones caused their breast cancer. These cases are slowly working their way through the court system.

What did the drug companies do after this? They kept selling, but attached new warning labels, like this one. This only added to women's confusion and fear, when looking for a solution to their symptoms:

## PREMARIN'S WARNING LABEL

### ESTROGENS HAVE BEEN REPORTED TO INCREASE THE RISK OF ENDOMETRIAL CARCINOMA

Three independent, case-controlled studies have reported an increased risk of endometrial cancer in post-menopausal women exposed to exogenous estrogens for more than one year. The risk was independent of the other known risk factors for endometrial cancer. These studies are further supported by the finding that incidence rates of endometrial cancer have increased sharply since 1969 in eight different areas of the United States with population-based cancer-reporting systems, an increase which may be related to the rapidly expanding use of estrogens during the last decade. *The three case-controlled studies reported that the risk of endometrial cancer in estrogen users was about 4.5 to 13.9 times greater than in nonusers* [my emphasis]. The risk appears to depend on both duration of treatments and on estrogen dose. In view of these findings, when estrogens are used for the treatment of menopausal symptoms, the lowest dose that will control symptoms should be utilized, and medication should be discontinued as soon as possible. When prolonged treatment is medically indicated, the patient should be re-assessed, on at least a semi-annual basis, to determine the need for continued therapy. Although the evidence must be considered prelimi-nary, one study suggests that cyclic administration of low doses of es-trogen may carry less risk than continuous administration. It therefore appears prudent to utilize such a regimen. Close clinical surveillance of all women taking estrogens is important. In all cases of undiagnosed persistent or recurring abnormal vaginal bleeding, adequate diagnos-tic measures should be undertaken to rule out malignancy. There is no evidence at present that natural estrogens are more or less hazardous than synthetic estrogens at equi-estrogenic doses.

According to Dr. Jonathan Wright, who pioneered the use of bioidentical hormone treatment in this country: "There are two key points in this warning: first taking Premarin for more than a year increases the risk of cancer of the endometrium as much as 14 percent. Well-controlled studies have shown that the risk of endometrial cancer is cumulative, rising at a rate of four to five cases per one thousand Premarin users with each year of use. By the fifth year of Premarin use, a woman might be facing a 2 percent risk and by her tenth year, her risk might be as high as 4 percent or 5 percent. Second: other forms of 'synthetic' estro-gen carry about the same risk."

What a dilemma. Synthetic hormones can *give* women cancer, yet today doctors still prescribe them. Not only are these synthetic drugs still prescribed, but they are often even used for frivolous purposes like treating acne (as well as to control breakthrough bleeding).

But what could a woman do? Most threw away their hormones and decided to go cold turkey. Women were suffering and feel-ing awful, but they were afraid of what these synthetic hormones could do to them and their health, and rightly so. That fear has likely carried over to you.

But around this time something great was also happening within medicine in this country. Western doctors were starting to learn about another approach to HRT: bioidenticals, or BHRT.

## BIOIDENTICAL HORMONE REPLACEMENT THERAPY (BHRT)

The information was out; synthetic hormones *are* dangerous, but enter bioidentical hormones! As you can imagine the drug companies were not happy about bioidenticals; synthetic hormones had been a twenty-billion-dollar-a-year business.

Natural bioidentical hormones are what our bodies make or once made. Hormones, as you know from earlier chapters, are essential to feeling good during this passage. So it makes sense to put back what is missing!

You may now be wondering: What makes bioidenticals different and safer than the horse urine pills?

The estrogen in conventional HRT is horse estrogen, not human estrogen. And progestin (medroxyprogesterone acetate) is not progesterone. This is a very important distinction. For example, bioidentical progesterone is made from a precursor compound found in wild yams or soy. They are then biochemically converted to molecules *identical* to human hormones. In short, they are *biologically identical* in their molecular structure to the human hormone, and as such are an exact chemical fit to what your body makes or once made.

That women still don't know about the benefits of these hormones is a travesty. It's due to a lack of doctor education, starting in our medical schools. Most medical schools receive funding from pharmaceutical companies to teach "allopathic medicine only," so the schools have a vested interest in training our new young doctors in the "pharmaceuticals are always best" school of thought, lest they lose their revenue stream. Sadly and unfortunately, when it comes to HRT, our students are taught a dangerous allopathic protocol, prescribing "one size fits all" doses of (what I call, fake) nonbioidentical hormones. This is where the bad rap and the confusion come in, making women wary of hormone replacement. How do you go against your doctor and his or her training? Clearly it is only with knowledge—that is the only thing that gives us the power to effect change.

Properly and artfully restored natural BHRT allows women (and men) to live a quality, healthy life (provided you take good diet and exercise seriously; there is no free lunch when it comes to your health and longevity).

## How BHRT Began

The very first doctor in the United States to prescribe a full course of BHRT was the brilliant maverick, the fearless Dr. Jonathan Wright. He found that by putting back what nature had once made, but in their purest forms, women were not only getting relief from menopausal (and perimenopausal) symptoms but they were enjoying better health overall. A new way was born.

Women started flocking to his practice, at the Tahoma Clinic, outside of Seattle, and Dr. Wright began teaching and training other doctors in the "art" of hormonal replacement. (He is one of the training doctors for ForeverHealth.com.)

The results were astounding: the use of bioidentical hormones produced an immediate decline in breast cancer rates of about 9 percent in his patients. I asked him to discuss how he came to this work, and how he discovered bioidentical hormones. Read what he had to say.

## BIOIDENTICAL TREATMENT:
## A PEEK UNDER THE HOOD

**JW:** To be accurate, I wasn't the first to discover them. It was Dr. John Lee who pioneered the use of bioidentical progesterone in the late 1970s. What I did, though, was to expand that use to a comprehensive program including estrogen, progesterone, DHEA, testosterone, thyroid, and even melatonin when needed.

From the time a female first enters puberty until the end of her last period all women are keenly aware of the constant hormonal changes going on inside their bodies. Except during the months of pregnancy, she will experience the complex ebbing and flowing of a twenty-eight-day cycle until she reaches her late forties or early fifties (and in some cases much earlier due to stress and toxicity). It's a natural and inevitable transition from one stage of life to another. Puberty marks the beginning of reproductive life, and menopause marks the end of it.

Even in the year 1050, bioidentical hormone replacement was being done very extensively in China, very similar to what we are doing today.

**SS:** Were they using soy and wild yams to make them?

**JW:** No, they were using human hormones extracted from the urine of young people who, of course, have the most hormones between the ages of fifteen and twenty-five. For the squeamish, urine has been used in medicine for years. Look at the drug Premarin, which is made from horse urine.

**SS:** Way back then they knew replacing hormones was beneficial?

**JW:** They were known as youth essence. The Chinese were also replacing hormones for the men, but it was limited to the emperor and his court. The "common people" did not get theirs. The physicians of the court were in charge of collecting, concentrating, and preparing the hormones from the urine, although at that time they didn't know they were collecting hormones; they just thought they were essences of youthful life.

**SS:** This was medication for the elite . . .

**JW:** Yes, for the elite in China. This went on from 1050 until the mid-1900s.

**SS:** Why did they stop using them? At present, hormones are a new concept in China. In fact, my book *The Sexy Years* only recently hit the book stands there and is selling quite vigorously.

**JW:** I don't have an explanation. Possibly, it's because the emperors had less and less power in the mid-1900s.

**SS:** How did you have the courage to begin prescribing them?

**JW:** Twenty-five years ago, one of my patients questioned the sanity of taking horse urine hormones. She didn't want them and gave me a challenge to find a way to make her feel better naturally. I knew at that time nutrition, good diet, vitamins and minerals, and some botanicals were crucially important, so I went to the textbooks and began at the beginning: What are estrogens in the body? What about progesterone? Then I started calling some of the very few compounding pharmacists that existed in North America in the early 1980s. I finally found a pharmacist, Ed Thorpe from Vancouver, British Columbia, who told me he thought he could source the molecular pattern. It took him about six weeks. And we started from there all because a patient came into my office and insisted that there had to be a better way, telling me she wasn't a horse!

**SS:** Good for her. How long did it take for her to start feeling well, and what did you give her?

**JW:** I've always believed in copying nature. I figured out what nature does and tried to use the exact same molecules in the exact same proportions and quantities that belong in the body. Plus, I tried to mimic the timing the body uses. The hormones I gave her at the time were the three classical estrogen hormones: estrone, estradiol, and estriol.

I did follow-up testing to make sure of its safety. I realized then that estrone wasn't essential in the formula, because estradiol turns into estrone on its own. I also made sure there was estriol in the formula because it is the anticarcinogenic component of the three estrogens. Estriol is very important in the makeup, but most doctors ignore or overlook this fact. Estriol is needed and here is why: it appears from a number of studies published over four decades that estriol's unique and most important role may be to oppose the growth of cancer, including cancer promoted by estradiol and estrone themselves. Animal studies show that when natural estradiol and estrone are "opposed" with estriol in normal physiologic proportions, the risk of cancer due to hormone replacement virtually vanishes.

**SS:** I've mentioned this in other books, but it was you that discovered my body doesn't make the estriol component of my estrogens, thus leaving me unprotected from cancer. I'm sure it's a big part of why I developed breast cancer, the other being a lack of progesterone, making me estrogen dominant. So I was really in trouble, no estriol protecting me as the anticancer component of my estrogens, too much estrogen in general, and no progesterone to oppose the estrogens. How many doctors could have figured this out?

You added estriol to my estrogen formula and I feel comforted that I am protected, and I am grateful for your understanding of the science of our hormonal selves.

In some form or another, natural hormones have been around in this country for about fifty years. But it wasn't until Dr. Wright had the courage to *prescribe* full BHRT in the United States over twenty-five years ago that women started to fully reap their benefits. He took such flack for his ideas about bioidenticals, yet bioidentical hormones reflect advances in physics and technology that simply were not available a half a century ago.

THE GOOD NEWS: The dangers of synthetic HRT do
not apply to state-of-the-art BHRT!

Bioidentical hormone replacement is safe, effective, different
from Premarin and Prempro, and proven beyond any reasonable
medical and scientific doubt.

These results were published in April 2007 in the *Journal of
the American Medical Association* and then again reinforced by
similar research published in the *New England Journal of Medicine* the following June.

## Why Isn't BHRT Standard Treatment?

Why hasn't the drug industry, knowing about synthetics and
their dangers, embraced bioidenticals more? Why haven't so
many heard about their safety and efficacy? The answer is that
hormones that occur naturally in the human body cannot be patented. A pharmaceutical company cannot own them exclusively.
No patent means less money! No patent means no pharmaceutical
company can have the exclusive right to manufacture and profit
from its product. Tremendous investment goes into developing
and studying a pharmaceutical product. It makes good business
sense for drug companies to protect their investment with exclusive patented products. As a result, there are also no double-blind
studies and minimal marketing of natural hormones.

To sell a drug, a pharmaceutical manufacturer instructs doctors on how and when to prescribe it. Much of what med students
are taught after university comes from pharmaceutical companies that have done extensive research in order to justify a product they sell.

When I urge replacement, I do not write about synthetic
hormones. I only write about natural bioidentical hormones
and BHRT. Bioidentical hormones can be individualized so

you receive the *exact* amount that your body is missing. Non-bioidentical hormones are "a one pill fits all" treatment with dangerous molecules. Why take synthetic hormones when natural hormones are better and safer?

Women have a powerful voice when used. Research and change is often initiated by informed patients like you, who have taken the time to learn, ask questions, and demand safer treatment options. Lately, the insistence of irate women has put pressure on some pharmaceutical companies to begin manufacturing natural hormones, but they are predosed. This means that if you get really lucky, possibly this particular formulation might be exactly what you need. What's more likely is that you'll "get close." In hormone replacement you don't want to get close. You want to find the perfect amount individualized just for you, to take away *all* your symptoms, not just some of them.

Because women have been so vocal about wanting natural hormones in the past few years, many doctors have started using pharmaceutical BHRT. Generally, they are not achieving the success that doctors who have embraced individualized dosing are having with compounded natural hormones.

Those who still argue the case for non-bioidentical hormones have an agenda, and usually this argument is made by a pharmaceutical rep who has a vested interest in promoting synthetics. They will argue that not enough research has been provided on the safety of natural hormones. Yet non-bioidentical hormones have been unequivocally proven to *give* patients cancer, stroke, and deep vein thrombosis! There is no data indicating that anyone has ever died using natural hormones. Bioidentical hormones do not have harmful side effects, if prescribed in the right dosages by a skilled doctor.

# FDA-APPROVED BIOIDENTICAL PRODUCTS

"Bioidentical" is a marketing term that has no accepted medical meaning.

—*USA Today*

This incorrect, inaccurate, and misinformed quote written by an Associated Press medical writer was broadcast all over the news media. The article it came from tried to discredit bioidentical hormones as non-FDA approved, and not proven safe or effective. Yet doctors write millions of prescriptions yearly for non-FDA-approved medications as part of routine medical practice.

As stated above, there *are* FDA-approved bioidentical hormones. The following list of bioidentical hormones were approved between 1996 and 2002:

Alora: A form of estradiol made by Watson Labs

AndroGel: Natural testosterone made by Unimed/Abbott

Climara: A form of estradiol manufactured by Bayer

Crinone: A form of progesterone made by Columbia Labs

Esclim: Estradiol, made by Women's First Healthcare

Estrace: Estradiol, produced at Bristol-Myers Squibb

Estraderm: Estradiol, created by Novartis

Estring: Another form of estradiol made by Pharmacia & Upjohn

FemPatch: Estradiol, made by Parke Davis

Prometrium: A progesterone manufactured by Solvay Pharmaceuticals

Testim: A testosterone produced by Auxilium

Vivelle-dot: Estradiol, produced by Novartis

These pharmaceutical bioidenticals are a step in the right direction but have one big drawback in my estimation: they are not individualized for exactly what *you* might need. As I said, these formulas can get close. And maybe you'll get lucky and find one whose amount just happens to be exactly right for you. But that is rare.

I prefer to get my hormones made by reputable compounding pharmacies—ones that are independently certified as following good manufacturing practices.

I get my hormones compounded so that I get my hormones individualized, *just for me.* This allows me to achieve a perfect balance, just like Goldilocks again: not too much, not too little, *just right.*

All patients may not need replacement of every hormone, every patient has different needs, and every patient is unique. How do you find out what you need? Keep reading, as the next chapter covers bioidenticals in depth.

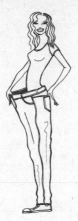

# CHAPTER 8

# BIOIDENTICAL HORMONES— THE GAME CHANGER

> The biggest human temptation is to settle for too little.
>
> —Thomas Merton

Many of us don't realize until we are well into perimenopause that the problem is hormonal decline. The bad moods are written off to stress, dissatisfaction with life, or our jobs . . . or close relationships. In many cases your children are starting to reach puberty at the same time that your hormones are declining. The collision of puberty and perimenopause within a household can feel like World War III.

I hear it all the time, "I'm too young for this!" Women see perimenopause as some sort of failure. Instead of being invincible, they are feeling out of control: the moods, the tears, the overwhelmed feelings. The reality is just nature at work . . . sadly accelerated by a major "push" from the environment.

Today's younger women have so much pressure. They feel like they have to do everything and do it perfectly. I call it, as have others, the "Superwoman syndrome." They do it all. They have perfect homes, perfect kids, perfect husbands, perfect hair, and perfect bodies. They excel at their careers, are on every important committee, and bring cupcakes (gluten free, of course) to school bake sales and parties. They juggle all their responsibilities and still find time to give perfect parties while wearing the perfect outfit.

Modern culture tells us this is what we are supposed to do and what we are supposed to be. It's written about in every magazine, every self-help book. When it doesn't work, we think we're somehow broken. What we should understand instead is that it's our hormones, not our failings. Until that reality hits we will continue to bark up the wrong tree, trying to excuse or explain why we feel like such a mess.

If this is you, your dedication and hard work is admirable. Your children have benefited, your marriage has benefited, your company or work has benefited, but . . . it is also very stressful. That stress isn't helping you now. Today's women enter perimenopause younger than ever before due to stress and toxicity, and both are difficult to avoid. Now it's time to take care of *you*!

## WHAT'S THE ANSWER?

There is no simple answer to perimenopause. Your body is changing, and it's a ten-year decline. To do nothing about your symptoms is to allow the discomfort you are already experiencing to accelerate, and never rectify the conditions associated with this transition. Your job at this point is to pay attention to your symptoms and find a doctor who can help you find balance. That is the point of this chapter: to provide you with all the information you need to have a well-informed conversation with a qualified doctor as you travel through this transition. There are many reasons and opposing forces working against you that add to the complexity of your declining hormones. All factors have to be considered if you are to expect optimal success in your personal regimen. Your best bet, in making this a smooth and enjoyable passage, is to replace the hormones you are steadily losing . . . but do so naturally.

I speak from experience. I was where you are today. From where I sit now—calm, sane, happy, healthy, blissfully enjoying life minute by minute, enjoying the loving relationship with my husband—I am here to tell you that I found my answer with bioidentical hormones and I've never looked back! Finding REAL natural bioidentical hormones to replace my almost nonexistent ones changed the course and quality of my life, as well as my work and life's mission. I was never in denial; I just didn't know what was happening to my body. I, too, thought I was too young. All I really knew then was that I just didn't feel right. And that was the understatement of the year.

Research has shown that after a woman's hormones start dropping, the earlier she begins supplementing her missing hormones, the healthier she will remain both short term and long term.

Ready to find out more, and maybe give BHRT a try?

## KNOW THE GOAL

The goal of natural hormone treatment is to bring the body back to balance, to replace what is missing, and bring the body back to your optimal healthy prime. Replacement alleviates the symptoms caused by the decline in the body's hormone production by using physiologic doses individualized for each woman. What I need is different from what you need. My stress levels are very high with my particular career so my needs are for larger amounts of estrogen, progesterone, and testosterone. Being "on" for a living can be quite stressful. Joyous stress, but stress just the same.

The goal of replacing missing hormones is to bring you to perfect balance, thereby giving you back your quality of life and in many cases (like mine) making you feel better than you've ever felt in your entire life.

## WITH TREATMENT—AS WITH LIFE— BALANCE IS KEY

Let's recap some of what you learned earlier about estrogen and progesterone in context with BHRT treatment. Here's the science.

Minor or sporadic fluctuations in levels of estrogen and progesterone have profound effects on your essential biological functions. Progesterone receptors are found throughout your body in most of the same areas as estrogen receptors, confirming the close, reciprocal relationship between the two.

Estrogen tells our cells to grow during the first part of the menstrual cycle, allowing for continual replenishment of old cells with new. Then progesterone steps in to redirect them, stopping cell growth. When the balance is off between the two hormones, you become symptomatic: your periods change, you can't sleep, you gain weight, you become forgetful and depressed. Your body tries to right things, but the fluctuations in perimenopause are erratic. Your body tries to stimulate ovulation, but you are alternating between high and low estrogen levels. These imbalances cause problems that are compounded when some months ovulation doesn't occur, and progesterone isn't produced.

Since estrogen is critical to your feeling of well-being, you might think the more you produce, the better you'll feel, but actually the opposite is true. In reality, drastic swings in estrogen levels make you feel worse and they also disrupt progesterone production. *It's the balance between estrogen and progesterone that is the key to feeling good during hormone transition.*

If your estrogen levels decrease gradually and maintain the same ratio to progesterone, you'll have a much easier time transitioning and fewer symptoms. When the shift is way out of balance, it generally causes unpleasant symptoms like irregular cycles, excessive bleeding, and bad moods!

We are each unique individuals. That's the beauty of each one of us. But every person has different hormonal requirements. That's why there is no "one pill fits all" in BHRT. Your hormonal requirements must be individualized, just for you. A qualified doctor understands this and works with you as an individual to tweak your dose until you hit the "sweet spot." When you hit that place of bliss, you suddenly remember what it used to be like all the time. This is what you will be striving for, and do know that you will achieve nirvana as long as you stay with it. I feel great . . . all the time. I have *NO* symptoms. I am sixty-six. If I can do it, so can you!

You will feel better almost immediately when you start replacement. It may take up to a full year, though, to get to the exact perfect place just for you. That is why I say over and over, patience is the key to achieving success.

# GETTING STARTED IS AS EASY AS 1-2-3

## Step 1: Find a Qualified Doctor

The first step is to find a qualified doctor. Replacing hormones naturally is a scientific art. You MUST find a qualified doctor who understands. If your doctor isn't prescribing bioidentical hormones, he or she likely needs to go back to school to learn about this form of treatment that wasn't taught in medical school. Currently, our medical schools give students approximately four hours of instruction on prescribing hormones. You will spend more time studying the art of replacing your hormones from having read this book than a premed student. Trust your new-found knowledge.

I highly recommend ForeverHealth.com as the site to find a vetted, qualified doctor nearest you. The service is free.

## Step 2: Write Down Your Symptoms

Before your appointment, write down your symptoms. What is your body saying to you? Remember these symptoms are not to be "toughed out." The longer you wait to do something about this body "language," the longer you will suffer. And I cannot stress enough, it is healthy to be hormonally *balanced. Imbalance* is *not* healthy and it's uncomfortable. Finding the source of these symptoms and correcting for them early on in perimenopause will allow you to sail through menopause.

You have a great advantage to be starting replacement this early on. With a good diet and exercise, a woman on BHRT can expect to feel good for the rest of her life. List everything you are experiencing. It won't seem stupid to a hormone doctor to tell him or her that your leg itches or that your vagina is dry. They "get" what your body is saying. Just discussing your symptoms with a *qualified* doctor will begin to assure you that it's all going to be okay. Once you have started replacement and are experiencing some alleviation of your symptoms, then the art part of replacement will begin.

## Step 3: Individualize Treatment

If you are still reading, you probably want to initiate an individualized bioidentical hormone program fast! The most efficient way of accomplishing this is to have a comprehensive blood test done even *before* your first doctor's visit.

The people at Life Extension offer a unique service where you can call them twenty-four hours a day at 1-888-718-5433 and order a Female Hormone Blood Test Panel. They immediately send out a requisition and location of blood drawing stations in your area. In most cases you'll get your results back within a week. (You can review the test in the resource section at the end of this book under "Getting Tested.")

Armed with your blood hormone readings, your doctor can immediately prescribe "starter hormones" to address your hormonal deficiencies. You will likely experience rapid relief of perimenopausal symptoms. If not, your doctor can order additional tests to fine-tune your bioidentical program so you can achieve a perfect, youthful balance. The art of BHRT is in its individualization. If you are young, you might just need progesterone replacement at first. If you are my age (sixty-six), you likely need the whole deal: estrogen, progesterone, testosterone, pregnenolone, DHEA, thyroid, adrenal output, and cortisol levels.

## PUT IT TO THE TEST—
## WHY BLOOD TESTING IS IMPORTANT

It's crucial to test your blood hormone levels so your doctor can initiate a customized bioidentical hormone program that's just right for you.

After you are placed on bioidentical hormones, some doctors (including Dr. Wright) will suggest a urine test that monitors the amount of estrogen and other hormones you are making over a twenty-four-hour period to get a more accurate picture of where you are hormonally. The first step is to identify your baseline hormone status. This is to know the ranges of all your hormones and gives you and your doctor the best picture for your symptoms.

You can take your blood test results to your current doctor, if you believe he or she is open to and skilled at this type of treatment. Or as I've said before, you can find a qualified doctor near you at ForeverHealth.com. Forever Health's doctors have chosen to step out of Western medicines' "standard of care" box and specialize in bioidentical hormone replacement. These doctors are also specializing in managing the changes that happen to aging bodies.

If you suspect you are entering perimenopause, it is extremely important to test your hormone levels. I asked Bill Faloon, founder of the Life Extension Foundation, an organization dedicated to keeping their members healthy and long-lived, to briefly explain why. My question to him was if a woman concludes that she is symptomatic and her decline has begun, should she get hormones replaced without testing her hormone levels? He replied:

"Think about this. . . . Would you drive your car without being able to see outside the windshield? That, regrettably, is how most conventional doctors treat their patients' problems. When a woman complains of symptoms related to sex hormone deficiency, if she's not with a qualified doctor, he may prescribe the same dose of estrogen, and possibly a synthetic progestin drug. The doctor hopes this blindly prescribed dose will alleviate perimenopausal symptoms. In other cases, the physician may not recognize the symptoms as being a hormone deficit and instead prescribes side-effect-laden antidepressant drugs, addictive antianxiety drugs, and/or sleeping pills.

"But with blood test results in hand, a qualified physician can determine the best individualized dose of natural estrogen, natural progesterone, DHEA, and other hormones required for preservation of healthy vitality."

Your exact needs for replacement will be determined by your lab results, as well as your complaints. If you are not sleeping, then your balance is not right. If you have no sex drive, then your balance is not right. You will get to that sweet spot, to your place of balance. This phase takes patience. DON'T GIVE UP!

Once your lab work is established, there are options in how you will replace your particular hormones. Your age is a factor. Often in perimenopause you are estrogen dominant, which as I said earlier means you are not making enough progesterone, so you have *excess* estrogen. This is not a good place to be.

Your blood tests will show if this is your scenario. Frequently, in the beginning of perimenopause, a little progesterone cream daily is all you need to get back to your old self again. By using it, you also protect yourself from the cancers that are allowed to proliferate from estrogen dominance.

## STATIC DOSING VERSUS RHYTHMIC CYCLING

Once your hormone levels have been established and you need more than just progesterone, as I did, you have two options: static dosing or rhythmic cycling. I believe that the two different methods work best according to the age and life stressors of the woman. For instance, a younger woman with ovaries is still making some hormone, and static dosing would be sufficient. Think of it as "filling the tank." She is simply going to need enough hormone to "top off" what she is already making in her own body. Her body is still making a "rhythm" (more on this later). An older woman such as myself (although I don't think of myself as old) is no longer making any hormones. I need to take my hormones in a rhythm to replicate what my body was making when I was young and fertile.

Let's start first with static dosing.

## Static Dosing

> Static dosing is taking the same amount of estrogen every day of the month and the same amount of progesterone for two weeks of each month. This creates a cycle that ends in a period each month.

To understand what I mean about age determining your choice in methods of replacement, I have been using BHRT for sixteen years. Initially, I was on static dosing. I was around fifty when I started on replacement. Knowing what I know now I should have been on replacement ten years earlier. Life would have been a lot easier, I probably wouldn't have gotten cancer, and I would have been a lot thinner and happier. (Thank you, Alan, for hanging in there with me.)

At that time, my body was still making some hormone but not enough to create a monthly estrogen peak. Because my body was still pumping out some estrogen hormone, I was able to fill in the gaps with replacement and still create a "peak" without realizing it. My body was still making some estrogen so by adding in enough bioidentical estrogen I could feel "right." I reached an estrogen peak, which allowed for the estrogen receptor sites to open to take in the progesterone on the eighteenth day.

Once your symptoms are discussed and their source determined, your doctor will prescribe the right amount of bioidentical estrogen every day (static dose) of the month. On days 18 to 28, your doctor will add in a static dose of progesterone based upon your lab work. This regimen is designed to match what our bodies once did when we were making a full complement of hormones. It brings about a period at the end of each cycle (at the end of the month). This approach is used because this is how it happens in nature, we have a twenty-eight-day cycle when we are reproductive.

Once you are on static dosing, your doctor will order a new blood test after a couple of months. Or order a twenty-four-hour urine test to get a sense of your new hormone levels. Again, if you are still symptomatic, it's important to keep track of your symptoms. It is the only way your doctor can truly know if the dosage is right for you. You know your body better than any lab test.

Many cutting-edge Western doctors (but not all of them) create this type of cycle with a period, in order to exactly replicate nature. Based upon the research I have done and information from the dozens of doctors I have interviewed, I will state firmly that I believe that cycling in this fashion is not an option, but a necessity. If we are trying to mimic normal physiology, this is the way to go.

## "DO I REALLY HAVE TO HAVE MY PERIOD TILL I'M NINETY?"

Dr. Jonathan Wright, the physician we discussed earlier who pioneered full BHRT usage in the United States, reports of a study that says that creating a period makes no difference. According to Dr. Wright:

Though I always say that to copy nature is the way to go, nature's plan is few to no ovarian steroids—bioidentical or otherwise—after menopause. But in the twenty-first century, with all of the changes of "civilization," that path leads to Alzheimer's, heart attack, stroke, and osteoporosis. So we've turned to nature's tools and used them very carefully, to prevent those problems. By having monthly bleeding cycles, we adhered to nature's plan. However, the very, very large majority of women have been asking since day one of my prescribing BHRT if it's absolutely necessary to have menstrual periods until they're ninety-one to avoid cancer risk. At first, I told 'em there was no research on this point, but if they really wanted—and most did—to avoid monthly bleeding and stay as safe as possible from cancer they must "take a break" every month. Then test at intervals for pro- and anticarcinogenic metabolites and predictive ratios of estrogens. Fortunately, doing this, not one woman I've worked with using BHRT has developed an estrogen-related cancer!

David Meyer's work came along in 1993 showing that a bleeding cycle is not necessary to prevent cancer. Nature is smarter than we are and has been using monthly menstrual bleeding for something else that we've learned about only recently: preventing women from having heart attacks and strokes! Menstrual bleeding reduces blood viscosity (thickness). Excess blood viscosity is the major cause of arterial wall damage that leads to inflammation, plaque formation, and ultimately heart attack and stroke. That's why menstruating women who don't take birth control pills or smoke cigarettes rarely if ever have heart attack. For men, heart attack risk may be reduced by 88 percent [see Salonen] and stroke risk may be reduced by 67 percent [see Meyers] just by donating blood once or twice yearly! Same applies to postmenopausal women, although no extensive research has been done.

Since this information became available, I have mentioned it to every woman asking for BHRT—and the very large majority tell me they'd rather donate blood twice yearly than have monthly bleeding. A small percentage decide to have monthly bleeding cycles. With blood donation, they're accomplishing a lot—if not nearly all—of what nature intended with monthly blood loss. So a lot of the why for not heavily promoting bleeding cycles has been for me adhering to women's personal choices. This information applies to postmenopausal women—those who no longer have a period—not to perimenopausal women. This is information for perimenopausal women to know for the next transition. I do push the large majority of postmenopausal women who make the "no period" choice to donate blood regularly and, in that way, copy nature!

Static dosing sounds simple, but there is a complex part. Stress affects and blunts hormone production. So if you are going through a stressful period in your life (and who isn't?), it changes your hormonal needs. To compensate, you may need to dose up a drop or a fraction of a milligram, or even lower your doses. If the stress is severe, you may need to have another blood test to determine where your levels are now.

This is another example of what I mean by the "art form" I mentioned earlier. It is important that you work closely with your doctor and communicate your symptoms so he or she will adjust your dosages until you get it just right.

When you are a perimenopausal woman, it can be difficult to accurately measure your hormone levels because they fluctuate so much, especially in the few years before menopause. You could measure your hormones three times in one day and get drastically different readings each time. That's nothing to panic about. Frankly, perimenopause is more difficult than menopause from my experience. Once you are in menopause, the body is drained of the minor hormones, so then replacement gets easier.

## Rhythmic Cycling

The second way to replace hormones is rhythmic cycling. I believe women of my age do best on rhythmic because we do not make any or very few sex hormones. It's actually a simple concept. It is once again mimicking nature. In other words, you are creating hormonal peaks through replacement just as when you were making a full hormonal complement on your own. For women who are drastically depleted, those whose bodies are not making any hormones at all or almost none, this puts you back together nicely, creating an estrogen peak each month by increasing and decreasing certain of your hormones.

You need to work closely with your qualified doctor at first.

It will require you to look at your monthly calendar daily and determine how much you need to apply/take each particular day. Again, the object is to create an estrogen peak, meaning that the highest amount of estrogen you take each month is on the twelfth day (when there is a full moon, as women's cycles have always been affected by the lunar cycle). Then it drops drastically on the thirteenth day. On the thirteenth day, you add progesterone in, and it keeps increasing until it reaches its peak.

Remember when your cycle was regular that there were days when you felt light and days you felt heavier, bluer? Remember days when you were feeling elated and days when you were feeling low? That was the rhythm you were making on your own. When you replace your hormones rhythmically, you don't have moody days (unless you are terribly stressed) because you can learn how to dose yourself a little higher or lower and in this way control and determine how you feel.

You won't take too much estrogen or progesterone because that in itself is uncomfortable and possibly you'll gain weight. If you are taking too much progesterone, you will bloat or get sleepy and lethargic. If you take too much testosterone, you will feel aggressive and grow chin hairs. (Nice, huh?) If you take too much thyroid, you will get a racing heart. You will learn. When it comes to being thin, vibrant, healthy, and sexual, we are motivated to learn fast!

Rhythmic cycling is based upon the ancient cycles of nature. This concept goes all the way back to early humans, who were attuned to the planet in a way that has become completely inaccessible to us in the modern world.

In the days of early humans, there were no executives or career women, just people living in tune with the cycles of the moon and the tides, reproducing as often as was possible. Each baby occupied a year of a woman's life, followed by breast-feeding for another couple of years. Interesting that we women reach our estrogen peak on the twelfth day, which is the full moon. As I explained in my book *Ageless*, if you go back to early humans when there was no light, couples could make love "by the light of the moon" on the day the woman was her most fertile. (Men should take notice and take us out to dinner on the full moon!) Women menstruated to the cycles of the moon, and we fattened up in the summer with all the abundant food. Then winter arrived and darkness came earlier. We went to sleep earlier because there was no light and we could stay warm with one another. Women's bellies grew with the baby made during the summer months. With spring we gave birth. Then the sun began to shine and the process started all over again. Simple! This was nature working at optimum before we got involved and messed with it.

When electricity came, it was declared a miracle, but it also changed our rhythms. Now we could stay up as late as we wanted. Without the proper amount of sleep, the work of all the healing hormones that normally happened from getting enough sleep each night was disrupted. So we slept less. Stress became a part of our lives and blunted our hormone production. We stopped cycling to the lunar calendar, we had fewer children, we breast-fed less, and in general we became weaker as a species.

Rhythmic cycling exactly mimics our healthiest prime, which would be us when we were our reproductive selves, when our hormones would rise and fall in peaks . . . a rhythm. Without a rhythm, the body perceives things as "not exactly right for reproduction," and it is in this imbalanced state that disease cells can begin to go wonky. Mimicking nature is the best way we can protect ourselves to avoid cell proliferation (cancer) and in turn keep organs intact as long as the rest of our diet and lifestyle habits are healthy.

Rhythmic cycling is worth looking into. It resonates. It makes sense. We do ebb and flow as human beings with the moon and the tides. It would make sense that our cycles would do the same.

Now that I am sixty-six, I do not make any sex hormones on my own anymore. None. So in order to create the right rhythm, I feel best at this time in my life taking my hormones in this way. I can't imagine how I'd feel or look had I not been replacing hormones all these years. I look at contemporaries who are afraid from lack of knowledge or who have a doctor who does not have the knowledge and they are not enjoying the kind of quality of life I have. Hormones make you happy. If you eat right and work out to some degree while replacing hormones, life and aging is a breeze. I enjoy every day.

## CONTINUOUS COMBINED HORMONE THERAPY

There is another way that doctors are prescribing BHRT: continuous combined hormone therapy. This means that you get a continuous combination of estrogen and progesterone, the same amount of both every day of the month.

Personally, I am not a proponent of this therapy. But I am not a doctor. Recent research out of Norway, analyzing data from 133,744 women, showed that these regimens confer a 43 percent greater risk of breast cancer (*see* Bakken).

Many women choose this protocol so they do not have to bother having a period. Talk to your doctor about the wisdom of mimicking pregnancy, and then make your own decision. Women on continuous combined do feel somewhat better because they are taking bioidentical hormones, and their symptoms are alleviated somewhat. But nature didn't ever give a women estrogen every day and progesterone every day unless she was pregnant. This would not be my personal choice. I don't believe a woman was meant to be pregnant or mimic pregnancy for the rest of her life.

## WHAT'S RIGHT FOR YOU?

Originally, I started on static dosing, but a few years ago I switched to rhythmic. It's whatever appeals to you.

It sounds complicated, but it really is as simple as looking at the calendar that accompanies your prescription. You look at the date of the month, and it shows you what amount to take that day. That's all it is. The thinking has been done for you.

Some women love how they feel on rhythmic and other women feel it is too much work and stop the protocol and go back to static dosing. It's all about feeling well, not having symptoms, what works for you, and what makes you the healthiest.

## BEFORE YOU GET STARTED— SOME BASICS

Women often ask me the same general questions about the basics of taking hormones. The rest of this chapter focuses on answering those questions. In addition, my trusted experts answer very specific questions on BHRT from women just like you in chapter 10, "Ask the Doctors—Real Questions, Real Answers."

### How Do I Take BHRT?

When your doctor prescribes BHRT, your compounding pharmacist will prepare for you exactly what *you* need. Hormones are usually taken through the skin, or transdermally, as a patch, gel, spray, or cream. This duplicates the way sex hormones are delivered in the body. Our endocrine hormones are absorbed directly into the bloodstream rather than through the digestive tract and the liver. This is another reason why taking bioidenticals orally (by mouth) is not optimal. Hormones taken orally must be processed by the liver, which can result in an increased incidence of blood clots and other related risks. Our livers are already so overloaded trying to eliminate environmental toxins. By taking them transdermally they not only don't cause clotting, but they are more effective.

### Isn't It Costly?

This is one of the top questions I hear: How much does it cost? The monthly cost of BHRT is not where the expense lies. The lab work to determine your deficiencies and needs, and the initial office visit to your qualified doctor, is the most expensive part. Insurance companies often won't cover expenses associated with women buying natural hormones (though some do). Not to sound like a broken record, if you go to ForeverHealth.com you will find a qualified doctor with an affordable office visit rate. After that initial visit and lab work, the price can range, but it's not outrageous. For instance, in my case where I am putting back all, my hormones run between $65 and $85 a month.

Until medicine shifts and insurance companies get more on board, only you can decide what you are willing to do, or even do without, to have the life quality and good health that these hormones provide.

### How Much Progesterone Should I Take?

Your qualified doctor will know how much progesterone to start you with and will increase the amount according to labs and your symptoms. Don't be afraid to dig deep and be specific on what's bothering you, so you can share it with your physician. Telling your doctor about every perimenopausal symptom is not being a hypochondriac. It's valuable information he or she can use to know how much or how little hormone treatment you need.

## What Type of Estrogen Should I Take?

BHRT is only available by prescription, prepared just for you at a compounding pharmacy. These pharmacies use only pure grades of estrogen. The strength and combinations of estrogens can be established by working closely with your doctor. Remember always: you know your body better than anyone. Some women require large doses to feel good. I am one of them. My body does not "sing" with low doses. Once you are on replacement, it is important to pay acute attention to how you are feeling and whether you are still experiencing symptoms. If you are still symptomatic, then you need to have your dosage evaluated. Talk to your doctor about it. A symptom might be as simple as mine: "my leg itches" (which can be a sign of low estrogen). Either way, replacing lost or declining estrogen with bioidentical estrogen will restore your body to your healthy prime.

## ARE YOU READY?

I've said it often in past books, and it always bears repeating: hormones are the "juice of youth." BHRT is real, natural, safe, and available. We are lucky to be alive at this time. Our daughters will certainly have an easier time of it because we've lighted the path. By the time they are grown up, I am convinced that BHRT will be the accepted way of dealing with perimenopause, menopause, and other symptoms of aging. We are the pioneers, and we are blazing the way for the next generation.

# CHAPTER 9

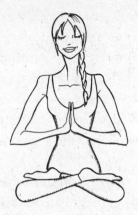

# HIDDEN FACTORS THAT COULD BE KEEPING YOU SYMPTOMATIC

*Life begins at the end of your comfort zone.*
—Neale Donald Walsch

If you are now on BHRT and still finding it hard to normalize, it could be food allergies and sensitivities, as well as other environmental factors. None of us can escape the environmental assault, so it's important to know how you might be affected and how it will hamper your efforts at health and hormonal balance. Read this section knowing that with knowledge you can survive the assault and find your ultimate sweet spot.

# IS YOUR FOOD HEALING OR HARMING?

An estimated thirty million Americans experience adverse reactions to foods such as dairy products, eggs, nuts, soybeans, wheat, and corn. Even when we don't think we are eating many of these foods, we may be consuming them in some form due to our overreliance on packaged and processed goods. For example, corn appears in many foods in the form of corn syrup and cornstarch. Casein, a milk protein, is used in breads, sauces, and baked goods.

Think of all the foods that fill our supermarket shelves and restaurants; how many of them have additives that did not come from nature? How many of these foods are genetically modified (GMO) or made up in chemical labs? Have you ever looked at the ingredients list for American cheese? It's not cheese at all, but a chemical look-alike concoction.

What are we thinking? No wonder our bodies are reacting violently. No wonder so many of us don't feel good. We have gotten so far away from the hunter-gatherer diets of early humans. Their diet was succulent roots and shoots, berries, leafy foliage, wild game, and foods that rotated with the seasons.

Unfortunately, today, it appears our bodies have not adapted to the monotonous, pesticide-riddled, chemically injected, non-nutritious foods of modern civilization. The air we breathe, the water we drink, and the food we eat determines our health and our quality of life.

## IS THIS YOU?

Do you have headaches, sinusitis, nasal stuffiness, heartburn, irritable bowel syndrome (IBS), muscle aches and stiffness, joint pain, anxiety, depression, difficulty sleeping, fatigue, skin itching, inability to focus, palpitations, or mental confusion? You could have food allergies. As many as 60 percent of people suffer from undetected food allergies with varied symptoms like the preceding.

There are two main food allergies: IgE (immunoglobulin E) and IgG (immunoglobulin G). People with IgE have reactions to things like peanuts or bee stings. The reaction can be immediate or occur a few hours after exposure. Reactions include hives, swelling around the mouth, asthma, diarrhea, vomiting, and even life-threatening anaphylaxis, a severe adverse reaction involving the major body systems. IgG (immunoglobulin G) is associated with delayed food reactions. The most common food offenders are milk, eggs, soy, and wheat. I happen to be allergic to eggs, cashews, and oftentimes dairy. If I eat these foods, I am wiped out, dog tired, and bloated, and my face puffs up like a balloon. Eating foods to which you are allergic or sensitive causes your immune system to attack you, just like it would a bacteria or virus; it's trying to protect you from the offending food. For people with sensitivities (depending on the degree) the smallest bit of the offending food can cause a reaction like say, a minispoonful of poison. Who would feel well taking any amount of poison?

Many people have food sensitivities and have no idea this is their problem. Something you ate four days ago may be causing today's migraine. So many suffer for years with chronic illness and symptoms never realizing that these conditions may be caused by something they are eating to which they are allergic or intolerant. When eating foods to which we are intolerant, inflammation takes hold in our bodies. That inflammation keeps us from being able to properly absorb the nutrients from our food. Being able to absorb your food is also critical in how well you age. Even if you are replacing hormones with bioidenticals, if your GI tract is inflamed, you will not be able to achieve balance. To have a balanced body, great health, and balanced hormones you have to look to your gut. If your gut is inflamed and unhealthy, nothing is going to work correctly.

I keep trying to test my body to be sure that it doesn't want eggs or dairy or cashews. It was very clear to me the other day when I had my once-a-year "date milkshake" that my body didn't like it. It tasted *so* good. Yet before I even finished, my stomach bloated up with gas and was uncomfortable for two days. I think my date-shake days are over! At least my body was clear with me; it did not want that milkshake.

Other foods you may be sensitive to may cause a delayed reaction, and therefore it can be difficult to associate the food with the symptoms it creates. Two things you can try immediately, if this is you: eliminate gluten and dairy for a couple of weeks to see how your body reacts. These are two of the most common intolerances, and well worth trying if you are suffering.

My husband, Alan, took years to realize his malaise, bloating, and fatigue was associated with gluten intolerance. As a result his testosterone levels plummeted, and even with replacement it wasn't doing the job until he made the connection—it was gluten. He had been eating organic food, was replacing his hormones, took supplements, did everything right, but still didn't feel "right." His stomach bloated every afternoon around three o'clock and he would have to take a nap from exhaustion. He would sleep eight to nine hours and wake up exhausted. Finally one of his tests came back and there it was: serious gluten intolerance.

He gave up gluten and everything normalized. He is no longer exhausted in the middle of the afternoon, he lost three inches off his waist, and his love handles disappeared. His food intake dropped in half (he did not realize he was eating double the amount of food he needed because the gluten problem did not permit the proper absorption of nutrients). Once he stopped gluten, his life and outlook changed. His hormone levels normalized with replacement, because now he could absorb them and his receptor sites received the messages to provide him hormonal balance.

If you suspect you are allergic to food or foods, or intolerant to specific foods, there are tests you can take to determine your intolerances. This important step could be the tipping point for you in getting to your ideal hormonal balance point if hormone replacement doesn't seem to be working for you.

A simple blood test is available. (Go to SuzanneSomers.com and click on Life Extension, or look at the Resources in the back of this book. Life Extension offers this test at a reasonable price and will interpret the results for you.)

Again, circling back, if you are using BHRT and not feeling great yet, food allergies just might be the obstacles that keep you from finding bliss. They are often the missing link to achieving balance.

It's difficult to balance hormones when you are breathing, eating, or drinking foods, poisons, and substances that are toxic to your body. That's up next: the toxins that can be keeping you "off."

## IS YOUR MATTRESS MAKING YOU FAT— AND SICK?

Most of us are now aware that we are exposed to toxins in our food, water, and air; however, we may not fully understand how many hidden ones we are surrounded by that we're not accounting for.

In her book *Silent Spring*, Rachel Carson writes, "For the first time in the history of the world, every human being is now subjected to contact with dangerous chemicals, from the moment of conception until death." That book was first written in 1962; imagine how many more dangerous toxins we are being exposed to today.

I asked Brenda Watson, author of *The Detox Strategy,* where else we are unknowingly taking in toxins. Her answer, which I shared with my readers in an earlier book, still bears repeating. It will shock you:

Let's begin with your bed. There are several ingredients that your body absorbs while you sleep, including toluene, a chemical linked to birth defects. It's emitted from the polyurethane foam that makes your bed so comfy. Then there's perfluorooctanoic acid, a chemical that makes fabrics stain resistant, but which is a hormone disrupter linked to ADHD in children. Next are the fire-retardant chemicals, some linked to learning disabilities and thyroid dysfunction, and some like antimony, linked to heart and lung problems. As of July 1, 2007, it was mandated by law that all mattresses manufactured or imported into the United States must be treated with these fire-retardant chemicals.

How about your carpet? Most likely it is synthetic and full of these same stain- and fire-resistant chemicals. When you brush your teeth, you know that warning label that says to keep your toothpaste out of reach of children under the age of six? Well, this label exists because your toothpaste exposes you to sodium fluoride, which is linked to enzyme disruption and thyroid problems. Also in your toothpaste may be sodium lauryl sulfate, which is linked to organ and reproductive (hormones) toxicity and triclosan, an antibacterial agent that's registered as a pesticide with the EPA and is linked to organ toxicity and possibly cancer. Most mouthwash contains formaldehyde and ammonia, several flavoring and coloring chemicals, as well as some chemicals that have leached from the plastic in the bottle.

Depending on the type of shampoo and soaps you are using, you expose yourself to coloring agents, dyes, artificial preservatives, and propylene glycol, a suspected carcinogen. Most antiperspirants contain aluminum zirconium, which is toxic to the nervous and reproductive systems; plus a chemical called BHT, believed to be a hormone disruptor and neurotoxin.

If you dry-clean your clothes, you are exposed to a plethora of chemicals, including perchloroethylene (PCE), a chemical believed to be capable of causing cancer, especially in the liver and kidneys. It is also shown to affect developing fetuses. Even if you don't get your clothes dry-cleaned, what about synthetic fibers in your clothing (think polyester), which may be giving off small molecules of plasticizer fumes?

It goes on and on. It's in your makeup, cosmetics, hair products, all of which are equally toxic. I don't write this to scare you. But to educate you as to why it's important to try to clean up your external environment while you seek hormonal balance during perimenopause.

You are dealing with two issues at perimenopause and both need to be considered seriously: declining hormones and the effects in your body from the changing toxic planet.

## STRESS IS TOXIC, TOO

You'll need to consider another issue, as it relates to that balance you are wanting: stress. It too is toxic, and it blunts hormone production. Don't forget to address it in your life and make lifestyle changes to lessen its hold. (Reread chapter 6, if you need some tips on doing so.)

Toxins in your food, on your food, toxins and hormones in the water, hormones and antibiotics in your meat, overuse of prescription drugs, toxic household cleaners, and even mold in your home—all can be can be reasons that your hormones are depleted prematurely. The brain is comprised of 65 percent fat. Mold and toxins love to hide in fat. This is dangerous for your brain. The brain also requires estrogen for neural replication, so if your brain gets toxic from the household cleaners or mold in your house, you can see how these dots connect and mess with your hormones. Detoxifying your house and your body will go a long way to ensuring good health—your body will thank you for it.

## STILL GAINING WEIGHT?
## SOMETHING NEW TO CONSIDER

The thyroid is specifically affected by toxins because many environmental chemicals have structures very similar to certain hormones and therefore are toxic to the thyroid. These chemicals can fit into the cellular receptors for these thyroid hormones with serious consequences, interfering with the usage and metabolism of the thyroid. When thyroid function is affected by these chemicals, it can't do its job of helping to normalize your metabolism. Without a functioning metabolism, you can't control weight gain.

Dr. Davis Lamson, of the Tahoma Clinic, has shown that toxic metals such as lead, mercury, cadmium, and many others can block the positive effects of thyroid hormone. (A chelation test will measure metal toxicity to determine if this is your issue.)

Fluoride, heavy metals, chemicals like perchlorates (found in drinking water), and x-rays can negatively affect the thyroid. Also certain medications damage or suppress thyroid function, including lithium, birth control pills, beta-blockers, phenytoin, antacids that contain aluminum, sulfa drugs, antihistamines, and chemotherapy drugs. Many of these same chemicals also mimic estrogen, testosterone, and other hormones like insulin.

This chemical assault now confuses the endocrine system, which is your hormone-making system. Remember if one hormone is off, all the hormones are off. Think back to the teeter-totter, except instead of the predictable low minors and high majors, with a chemical assault it's all wacky; chemical sensitivities might make the minors go high, and the majors low. Now your balance is off; either way, you will not feel well, your moods will be affected as will your weight and your libido, causing your entire body system to not feel "right." In addition, you'll be displaying symptoms such as sleeplessness, anger, body itches, stomach bloating, extreme fatigue, uncontrollable body temperatures (either too hot or too cold), memory lapses, and no sexual desire. A qualified doctor (visit ForeverHealth.com to find one in your area) specializing in natural BHRT and/or environmental medicine will understand how to detox these harmful chemicals out of you so you can achieve perfect balance again. By making the effort, you will be the winner.

For those who choose not to accept that the environment and stress are culprits blocking their opportunity for true health, their bodies will most likely continue to deplete hormonally at earlier and earlier ages. The hidden factors may be the reasons why it is harder for your body to accept hormone replacement and sadly, depletion sucks the life out of you. Don't let this happen. Our body talks to us all the time. Remember to pay attention to its language. For instance:

- If your eyes are puffy, you need to check your thyroid.
- If your shoulders feel tight and constricted constantly, you should test for human growth hormone. HGH positively affects lean muscle mass, keeping you fit and limber.
- If your skin is wrinkling prematurely or your muscles are lax, your estrogen levels may need adjusting. You may also have a deficiency in DHEA and HGH.
- If you are experiencing memory loss, you could be pregnenolone deficient.
- Estrogen depletion will also give you "foggy brain."

- Imbalanced thyroid, either high (hyperthyroid) or low (hypothyroid), will affect your ability to think straight.
- Adrenal fatigue also affects thinking and can cause a brain drain.

You can see that looking at one aspect, one absolute, like focusing on just one hormone, might not lead you to the culprit. It could be one or many causes that are wreaking the havoc.

There are many other signs and signals as identified throughout this book that our bodies give to each of us. Learning this language, what each sign and signal means, how each works, and what to do about it, is the purpose of this book. Use your newly acquired knowledge of perimenopause to your advantage and "hear" it.

## STAY THE COURSE

Continue to work with your doctor. Talk to him or her. Dig deeper. Your doctor can analyze your hormonal ratios to help you achieve optimum health. Amazingly, with today's new medical approaches, we can now test an individual's genetics and possibly circumvent issues long before a problem surfaces. "Genetically predisposed" does not have to be your fate. The new doctors can pinpoint your allergies, intolerances, and genetic factors to vastly improve your health and metabolism, plus they can test to see if mercury, lead, cadmium, heavy metals, or other new environmental substances are responsible for your diminishing health. This kind of detective work just might uncover causes for the conditions you are experiencing, for example, where did your autoimmune disease come from and why?

The new environmental doctors can test for molds and bacteria that slip into our bodies and wreak havoc. Your doctor can then determine how these issues can be rectified in order to restore you to optimum health and hormonal balance. The detective work continues: something as basic as your homocysteine level and finding it elevated could indicate future heart disease or determine that you are not detoxifying properly. Uncovering this could be another part of the puzzle as to what is making your hormones imbalanced. There are so many factors today and to properly serve patients it requires new thinking on the part of our doctors. Don't settle for less.

Our food has changed, our air and water are now mostly polluted, and the planet in general is not the same as it was fifty years ago. To find hormonal balance and quality of life will require diligence. But you can do it! Make changes in your diet, your environment, rethink your lifestyle, get proper sleep, manage your stress, and make sure you get sufficient exercise. These things seem simple but they are the game-changers separating those who can withstand the overwhelming assault and sail through perimenopause, from those who can't.

The new approach to health and our transitions is exciting detective work. We can now dig deeper than ever before to unravel the mysteries of body balance. It is equal parts back to basics and advanced science. But merging these two schools of thought is creating better quality of life for all of us. I emphasize repeatedly in this book to work with a doctor or doctors who understand the new way to stay healthy. If your doctor hasn't kept up, then find one who has.

> This cutting-edge approach to true health is the most exciting change in health care to come along in our lifetimes.

# DON'T GIVE UP!

Throughout the years I've heard women complain that they have tried hormone replacement but it didn't work for them. If this is you, dig deeper. Don't lose out on this progress in women's health. Get to the bottom of your hormonal puzzle. Don't give up until you feel *perfect*. You can and will!

Hormonal balance and all the joy that comes with it is yours with BHRT replacement, as long as you take all options into consideration. Your commitment to great health will pay off immeasurably for you *and* for your family. These are exciting times for women, much different from the women who came before us. You can get your life back with this new knowledge and embrace perimenopause knowing that you will emerge triumphantly as the vibrant, sexy, healthy, exciting, and happy woman you deserve to be!

CHAPTER 10

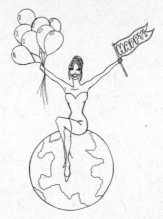

# ASK THE DOCTORS—REAL QUESTIONS, REAL ANSWERS

Women have so many questions when entering perimeno-pause. It takes a qualified doctor to help a woman navigate this difficult and confusing passage. I asked fourteen of the doctors at ForeverHealth.com to answer my readers' most common questions. Each of the doctors in the Forever Health Network has been vetted and trained to provide optimal, cutting-edge new medicine, including bioidentical hormone replacement therapy.

If you see yourself in these questions (or answers), these doctors and others at Forever Health will be able to help you find relief. Please first talk with your personal physician before attempting treatment or going it alone or better yet, go to Forever Health.com and connect with the doctor of your choice in your area. These doctors know what they are doing, they understand the changing planet, and they understand the effects of stress and toxicity on the hormonal system and how it affects each woman differently.

The contributors to this chapter include:

Dr. Sean Breen

Dr. Evelyn Brust

Dr. Rachel Burnett

Dr. Sue Decotiis

Dr. Gail Gagnon

Dr. Michael Galitzer

Dr. Prudence Hall

Dr. Anju Mathur

Dr. Marsha Nunley

Dr. Joseph Raffaele

Dr. Theresa Ramsey

Dr. Gowri Rocco

Dr. Ron Rothenberg

Dr. Neil Rouzier

All these doctors are at the top of their field and leaders in the new way to age with quality of life.

## PERIMENOPAUSE SYMPTOMS . . . ?

*Q: I am just beginning to see the signs of perimenopause kicking in. I don't want to lose my sex drive or vitality. Are there steps or hormones I can start taking now to avoid those issues? And are there other changes I can make in my diet and exercise to help, too?*

DR. MICHAEL GALITZER: Yes, there are plenty of things you can do. As far as diet is concerned: eat organic, and avoid wheat and dairy products. Eat high-quality protein at each meal, and take a multivitamin, 2,000 mg of vitamin C daily, and 4,000 IU vitamin D daily. Get a blood test for all your key hormones on day 20 or 21 of your menstrual cycle (first thing in the morning)— thyroid, cortisol, DHEA sulfate, estrogen, progesterone, testosterone, FSH, LH, and insulin. See a physician who is well versed in BHRT to assist you in balancing these hormones. Also, combine aerobic exercise with yoga and/or Pilates four times a week.

*Q: Are excessive bleeding, longer periods, and shorter duration between periods part of perimenopause? I take birth control pills to regulate my periods—would I be better off with bioidentical hormone therapy? How do I know if I am in perimenopause?*

DR. JOSEPH RAFFAELE: Perimenopause is defined as the four to six years (sometimes longer) before a woman has her last period. During this passage, your time between periods (your cycle length) can vary by more than seven days, both longer and shorter. So, if you have periods that vary by this much or if you miss more than two periods in your mid to late forties, then you are likely in perimenopause. If your doctor tests your FSH level and it is above 25 and you have these symptoms, then you are assuredly in perimenopause.

The shorter cycles usually occur because you are not making adequate progesterone during the second half of your cycle and that causes your uterine lining to shed off prematurely and sometimes very heavily. I usually treat this by adding progesterone on the fifteenth to twenty-eighth day of the cycle (day one being the first day of the period). Sometimes, not enough estradiol is made by the ovaries and you don't have enough lining to shed off so you can miss a period altogether, or it can happen late. If a woman has symptoms of estrogen deficiency such as brain fog, night sweats, and hot flushes, I add some estradiol to her regimen. At times, some women make more estrogen than they ever have and experience severe bloating, cramps, breast tenderness, and heavy bleeding. These women often benefit from daily progesterone to dampen the effects of the excessive estrogen production.

Birth control pills are commonly prescribed to perimenopausal women to control their irregular cycles and heavy bleeding. In most cases it does this quite well and is simple to do. But I *never* prescribe oral contraceptives to perimenopausal women. First, I can almost always get control of these symptoms in the ways described above, though I'll admit it can take a little more work to find the right combination and dose than just popping a pill out of a plastic dial. Second, and more important, the estrogen and the progestins in BCPs are not bioidentical and they can lower free testosterone, decrease the effectiveness of growth hormone secretion, increase the risk of blood clots, and expose your breasts to much higher levels of estrogen than is necessary. Gynecologists often counter that my recommendation puts the patient at risk of getting pregnant. True, there is a *small* chance that she may get pregnant, but that can be addressed by nonhormonal means and most patients agree that the convenience of the pill isn't worth the adverse effects.

*Q: I was told that I am in perimenopause. I'm thirty-nine years old. This was told to me by the acupuncture doctor. But my primary doctor says I'm "fine." I don't know what to believe. I don't feel like myself, I have anxiety, and I can't lose weight no matter what I do.*

DR. PRUDENCE HALL: Your question is one that frustrates me as well. Patients experiencing major symptoms of perimenopause constantly tell me that their hormones were "normal," per their doctors. They were then denied treatment. Many doctors simply don't even recognize that perimenopause exists, and if they do, aren't aware that it commonly begins in a woman's mid to late thirties and into her early forties. Because estradiol levels are frequently only slightly decreased on blood work at these ages, the deficiency is overlooked. The pituitary hormone goes above 20 in menopause, but in perimenopause is either totally normal or just slightly increased a bit beyond the normal 2 to 5 range. Doctors are so used to looking at lab values that we can forget to actually listen to what our patients are telling us. Perimenopausal patients tell us that they are tired, have worsening PMS, wake up in the middle of the night, are gaining weight for no reason, feel anxious and depressed, and are also quite irritable. A lowered sex drive also comes out of the blue, which is common with low estradiol states. When patients describe these symptoms, I usually prescribe a low dose of bioidentical estradiol at their PMS time, or all cycle long depending on what is needed, per their individual symptoms. In thousands of cases, patients feel normal again, and feel their symptoms reversed. Because low thyroid and adrenals can mimic many of these symptoms, I always do a panel to check all hormones and correct any hormone that is deficient, even if it is only slightly low.

*Q: I have been suffering through perimenopause for a year now. I turned fifty this past April and since then I feel like I'm falling apart! I am trying to find a natural hormone replacement doc in my area but I also know they can be expensive. What other natural steps can I take?*

DR. ANJU MATHUR: You sound like someone who really needs to get on bioidentical hormones as soon as possible. In the meantime, you can improve your diet to support optimal female hormone activity. Eat enough calories. Follow a Paleolithic diet: one that focuses on fruits, vegetables, meat, poultry, and fish. Add amino acid supplements and eat organic foods. Avoid caffeinated drinks, sugar, sweets, soda, cookies, bread, and pasta. Avoid grains and dairy products. Avoid being overweight. Avoid excessive chronic stress, Avoid cigarette smoking or any drugs.

## TESTOSTERONE DOSING

*Q: I want to know your thoughts about the general dosing schedule for bioidentical compounded testosterone. Is it generally the norm to apply the cream every day or should we take a few days off each month as is the case with progesterone?*

DR. MICHAEL GALITZER: Bioidentical testosterone is usually applied as a cream in a dose of 1–5 mg *every* morning depending on the results of a blood test for testosterone.

## MOOD SWINGS

*Q: I would love to know what I can do to alleviate my mood swings! I'm like Jekyll and Hyde!*

DR. PRUDENCE HALL: Mood Swings R Us should be the name of perimenopause and menopause. They are caused by a combination of fluctuating and declining estrogen, as well as the thyroid and adrenal glands becoming imbalanced. I am, of course, a big proponent of women rebalancing every hormone that becomes deficient back to a youthful, healthy level. This involves getting your hormone levels checked, as well as having your doctor prescribe bioidentical hormones to correct each deficiency. To help the rebalancing process along naturally, I suggest you begin Mark Whitwell's seven-minute daily, "The Promise Practice" [ThePromise.com]. It helps the natural healing forces of life to operate powerfully in you. Also get eight or nine hours of sleep, begin eating an anti-inflammatory diet (eliminating dairy, gluten, eggs, and soy), and take digestive and systemic enzymes.

## PMS OUT OF CONTROL

*Q: Why is my PMS getting worse?*

DR. MICHAEL GALITZER: Stress is the major reason for worsening PMS symptoms. The adrenal glands are the organs that have to secrete hormones in response to stress. With continued stress, the adrenal glands become depleted. They then draw from the ovarian hormones—estrogen and progesterone. Consequently, you get depleted of your ovarian hormones, and your PMS gets worse. Get a blood test for all your key hormones (DHEA, cortisol, thyroid, estrogen, progesterone, LH, and FSH) on day 21 of your menstrual cycle, and see a physician who is well versed in BHRT. The three supplements that are most helpful with PMS are zinc, vitamin $B_6$, and evening primrose oil.

*Q: I took birth control pills for twenty years and stopped a year ago. Since then I have experienced severe PMS, cramps, mood swings, etc. Working during this time every month is quite difficult. My husband says that I become possessed during this time. Once I start my period, then I'm fine. I'm ready to go back on the BCPs to control my PMS. What else can I do and will hormones help?*

DR. NEIL ROUZIER: Your PMS symptom complex is very common and needlessly suffered by many women like you. As you have experienced, there are times that you feel great and times that you can't stand it. Some women have no symptoms of PMS and others suffer terribly. Fortunately there is a very effective, safe, and healthy solution to your PMS: progesterone. It is the fall in your progesterone levels that is causing your symptoms. It is the fall in progesterone levels at delivery that results in postpartum depression. If you suffer from PMS, you may also be the one who encounters depression after delivery. Both are easily treated with progesterone.

In the past, I used to treat PMS by having women take progesterone just during the days of PMS, seven to ten days before their period. Patients would tell me that they did not stop the progesterone but continued to take it throughout their cycle because they felt better on the progesterone than off. I now treat with daily progesterone and increase it as needed on days of PMS. A common error in treating PMS is that many women do not use enough progesterone to control symptoms. One has to sometimes use high doses of progesterone, and only then will the symptoms of PMS be relieved. If you still have symptoms of PMS, then you are not taking enough progesterone.

## MIGRAINE AND OTHER HEADACHES

*Q: I am a migraine sufferer and this phase has been at times overwhelming. Is there any help?*

DR. MICHAEL GALITZER: Migraines may sometimes be a result of an overloaded liver, but there can be associated triggers such as food sensitivities, mercury toxicity from excessive ingestion of fish (such as tuna and swordfish), as well as the presence of silver amalgam fillings, and pesticides, to name a few of the environmental toxins that we are constantly exposed to.

Optimizing the health of your liver is paramount. You can do the following:

   1. Juice a lemon in six ounces of water first thing in the morning.

2. Increase your intake of carrots, beets, zucchini, squash, and artichokes.

3. Juice green vegetables daily.

4. Take specific liver herbs such as milk thistle daily.

5. Get a high-quality multivitamin

6. Take vitamin C (2,000 mg) twice a day.

7. See an acupuncturist.

8. Use an infrared sauna twice a week for thirty minutes at a time, drinking plenty of water while in the sauna.

Please get a blood test for all your hormones including: thyroid, DHEA sulfate, cortisol, estrogen, progesterone, FSH, and LH. You will most likely need supplementation with bioidentical estrogen and progesterone, by a physician well versed in this type of treatment.

*Q: I'm forty-seven and have been on bioidentical progesterone for ten years, and it's been wonderful. Lately, though, I have experienced bad headaches prior to my cycle. Is this a sign of me needing to start using estrogen also?*

DR. MARSHA NUNLEY: Possibly. It is likely that you are having increasing fluctuations in your hormones, particularly estrogen. The body prefers for things to be stable, so the hormone fluctuations of the perimenopausal period can bring on symptoms like headaches. It could also be related to adrenal or thyroid issues, and diet and lifestyle could be a contributing factor. Testosterone can drop significantly during perimenopause and replacement might be helpful. You may also need to increase the progesterone.

# FEAR OF CANCER

*Q: Will using BHRT cause cancer and is it safe? What about thermography for scans?*

DR. NEIL ROUZIER: Bioidentical hormones will not guarantee that you not get breast cancer. Cancer can be caused by genetic, environmental, lifestyle, and many yet to be discovered causes. Your question would require pages and pages to fully explain the difference in hormones, the protective effect of some and the harm of others. I will summarize this very complex and confusing topic. Thanks to the media sensationalism, most women (and physicians) are falsely led to believe that all hormones cause cancer, and this is simply not true. For years we have preached and taught that synthetic hormones can cause cancer, and it is well documented in scientific studies that medroxyprogesterone (Provera) increases the risk of cancer. The recent lawsuits against Wyeth are the result of this. The largest and most powerful study to date, the Women's Health Initiative (WHI) trial, proved that the combination of PremPro caused an increase in breast cancer incidence. Other recent studies utilizing estradiol and natural, bioidentical progesterone did not show any increased incidence in cancer. So the culprit seems to be the synthetic progestin (Provera) and not progesterone. Although estrogen may cause a cancer to grow once it becomes established (estrogen + receptor tumor), all data prove that estrogen does not cause the cancer to occur in the first place. Rest assured that the most recent powerful scientific studies do not support the theory that estrogen causes cancer.

Here is the most important part of your answer, however. There are multiple studies in the literature that prove natural progesterone is protective against cancer. The largest and longest study in the world, the EPIC-E3N study published in the journal

*Cancer,* has continuously demonstrated that addition of progesterone to estrogen decreases the incidence of breast cancer, whereas the addition of a synthetic progestin (Provera) does increase risk significantly. Multiple other studies demonstrate that progesterone does not increase the risk of cancer, yet Provera did. Multiple studies demonstrate that the higher your progesterone level is, the more down-regulation of breast tissues and protection against breast cancer, and this is through various mechanisms. Although many women falsely believe that natural estrogen is protective, it is actually the cancer-killing (apoptotic) effect of natural progesterone that is responsible for the protection against breast cancer. I hope this has cleared up any misconceptions about which hormones cause cancer (synthetic progestins), which ones protect against cancer (bioidentical progesterone), and which ones have a neutral effect (estrogen).

Thermography has become popular as a more benign, less painful alternative to mammography. Although modern mammograms are more accurate and sensitive due to advances in technology, thermography is another option that is painless and preferred by many who can't tolerate mammograms or have an aversion to them.

*Q: If you had breast cancer and thyroid cancer, is it okay to take hormone replacement? I believe my cancer came from taking Provera; after nine months, I took myself off but three months later I had a lump.*

DR. ANJU MATHUR: If your breast cancer was treated and you are cancer free at the moment, then hormones could be used with caution. I usually check twenty-four-hour urine tests to determine estrogen quotient, as well as 2/16 alpha-hydroxyestrone ratio. If they are abnormal, I treat them with natural supplements to lower the risk of recurrence. At the same time, every effort should be made to boost your immune system. Failure of the immune system likely caused the cancer cells to grow unchecked in the first place. Provera is a synthetic progesterone called progestin and it is connected to an increased risk of cancer.

*Q: Do bioidentical hormones increase your chances to get breast cancer?*

DR. RON ROTHENBERG: There have been many studies to show that BHRT does not increase your risk for cancer. Having said that, anyone can get cancer with or without hormones, so taking hormones does not give you immunity to developing cancer. The idea that hormone replacement increases the risk of breast cancer came from the Women's Health Initiative Study published in 2002. This flawed study produced a lot of confusion in physicians and in women in general. The drugs studied were Premarin or conjugated equine estrogens derived from horse urine (which is a very cruel process for us animal lovers) and Provera or MPA, which is artificial, chemically altered progesterone, not bioidentical progesterone. We now know that estrogens should always be bioidentical and administered through the skin with creams, gels, or patches, not taken orally. But even the orally given horse estrogen when used alone did not increase breast cancer risks.

The most dangerous component of "old school HRT" is the artificial nonbioidentical progestin, Provera or MPA. A study in France tracked 80,000 women who were using transdermal bioidentical estrogen and bioidentical progesterone versus estrogen and MPA (*see* Fournier). After eight years, the risk of breast cancer in the bioidentical estrogen and progesterone group was the same as the risk of a woman who had not taken any hormones. In the MPA or Provera group, there was a 69 percent increased risk of developing breast cancer.

Replacing deficient estrogen, progesterone, and testosterone at perimenopause and menopause with bioidentical hormones has significant quality of life benefits as well as protection of cardiovascular, cognitive, and sexual function, and preventing osteoporosis.

## NATURAL WAYS TO REGULATE HORMONES

*Q: Is there anything all natural that will help regulate your hormones? Or bring you to an equal median?*

DR. MARSHA NUNLEY: A low glycemic diet with lots of brightly colored and green vegetables along with a daily exercise program, adequate sleep, and a stress-free life can help. Herbal supplements to consider include black cohosh, chastetree berry, a rhubarb supplement (Metagenics makes a good one), and all may be somewhat helpful. Bottom line: nothing works as well as bioidentical hormones.

## ACNE

*Q: Adult acne! How to stop it?*

DR. SUE DECOTIIS: Adult acne is an unpleasant surprise for many adults who never had teenage acne. The chief underlying cause is hormonal imbalances that present symptoms in the form of acne. Too often the cycle of stress and overproduction of androgens and cortisol by the adrenal gland causes overproduction of oil by sebaceous glands of the skin. The ducts of these glands become clogged with bacteria and debris, which leads to acne. During the second half of the menstrual cycle, progesterone levels rise and fall quickly and estrogen levels remain low. So even normal levels of androgens remain unopposed due to these cyclical drops. This androgen dominance, be it ever so brief during the cycle, can also cause increased oil production and induce acne at this time. An antibacterial cleanser can be helpful for just about all acne sufferers. Traditionally adult acne has been treated by prescriptions of oral or topical antibiotics. Yet attacking the bacterial component of acne is merely treating a complication of the increased oil production. Hormone levels should be tested. Medicinal strength glycolic acid peels can also be helpful. If testosterone levels are elevated, an antiandrogen medication such as Spironolactone can often be effective. But trying to alleviate stress and reduce inflammation in the body is extremely important. Taking micronized omega-3 (fish oil) capsules as well as a medicinal-grade probiotic, avoiding refined carbohydrates such as starches and sugar, exercising, yoga, and meditation are all important steps. Stress is detrimental to general health and can affect every organ system. Learning to manage stress is key to your well-being as well as to clear skin. If there are other accompanying symptoms, such as excess hair growth, weight gain, menstrual irregularities, or headaches, your physician should look for other underlying causes.

## ITCHY SCALP

*Q: Is there a connection between perimenopause and an incredibly itchy scalp? I have seen a doctor and do not have dandruff or anything, yet nothing I do for it helps!!*

DR. SUE DECOTIIS: Dry skin and itchy scalp can be seen with estrogen deficiency. BHRT can help by returning the moisture in skin that estrogen helps maintain. More specifically, estriol, an estrogen, can be used specifically on the skin and on the scalp in a compounded formula. It is also important to check for thyroid deficiency, as this can be a cause of the symptoms. Don't over-look obvious causes such as fungal dermatitis, eczema, and psoriasis. In addition to topical estriol and BHRT, moisturizing oils such as jojoba, and vitamins such as folic acid, B complex, biotin, and DL methionine could help. In my practice I often pre-scribe a compounded mixture of estriol, alpha lipoic acid, and coenzyme $Q_{10}$. Vitamin C ester can promote a youthful glow to the skin, too.

## FEELING ANXIOUS

*Q: Could anxiety be a sign of a hormone imbalance? Is it common to suddenly develop anxiety in your early forties, without any of the other typical menopausal symptoms? And what hormone would be responsible for these anxious feelings?*

DR. SUE DECOTIIS: Anxiety is definitely a common symptom of perimenopause. It is often the first symptom to occur during the time that hormone levels are shifting. Progesterone levels can decline early on in the process, with estrogen levels staying the same. This leads to a relative "excess" of estrogen. Nervousness, irritability, moodiness, insomnia, and restlessness can all occur during this time. Anxiety can present along with other symp-toms due to this hormonal shift, which I explain to my patients as the "FIVE B's"—bitchiness, bloating, bleeding (abnormally heavy and or frequent periods), decreased libido, and breast ten-derness. Many women start experiencing weight gain during this time. Progesterone decline, which occurs transiently during the menstrual cycles of premenopausal women, is responsible for PMS, PMDD, and menstrual distress.

After checking hormone levels on the twenty-first day of the menstrual cycle, bioidentical progesterone can be prescribed.

After correcting this imbalance, patients report alleviation of the symptoms mentioned and feeling like themselves again. The perimenopausal period may last quite a long time. Not diagnosing the real problem and correcting the hormonal imbalance can make for a very traumatic time in a woman's life. Many perimenopausal women are treated for depression and insomnia, or see psychiatrists and marriage counselors, when an accurate diagnosis and treatment could avoid this.

## PANIC ATTACKS

*Q: Are panic attacks and anxiety part of perimenopause?*

DR. GOWRI ROCCO: Although most published symptoms of menopause do not usually include anxiety and/or panic attacks, these symptoms do get much worse or even start happening at the time of perimenopause. Women often complain of increased nervousness, irritability, unnecessary worrying, low resistance to stress, low confidence, and increased depression with lowering levels of progesterone. Rebalancing progesterone significantly reduces a lot of these symptoms, to the point that conventional drug treatments may not be needed for anxiety, depression, or sleep. L-theanine is an excellent supplement to take for decreasing anxiety after progesterone is rebalanced, and it also is a natural "chill pill" that has no addictive properties and hardly any side effects reported with even high dose use. I recommend 200 mg L-theanine as needed for anxiety, and 400 mg for panic attacks to my patients. L-theanine is also great for inducing calm and inducing sleep, especially if poor sleep is related to excessive thinking and worrying. L-theanine is an amino acid and has a short half-life, with no drowsiness effects when taken during the day.

*Q: When you're experiencing some unusual symptoms of anxious moments, when it has not occurred before, which hormones are most likely to be unbalanced? When do you take yourself to the M.D.?*

DR. PRUDENCE HALL: That is such a good question; the symptoms could actually point to a few imbalanced hormones. Anxiety and nervousness are common in perimenopause and can be symptomatic of hormone imbalance. The adrenal hormones are also frequently stressed, causing surges of anxiety. Symptoms are a good way to measure your hormonal decline. Hot flashes, night sweats, weight gain, depression and anxiety, and a decreasing sex drive all suggest you should check in with your doctor to have your hormone levels balanced.

## FEELING BLUE

*Q: I am forty-one and I am having more "blue" days than I have ever had. I am not depressed, but some days it sure seems like it. Is that normal?*

DR. JOSEPH RAFFAELE: There are many things that can cause an increase in the days a woman feels "blue." Difficult life events, stresses, and relationships can all contribute. These are the "normal" things that can build up and depress mood. By age forty-one, most women also have considerably lower testosterone levels than when they were in their twenties. The lower levels often leave women with less energy and "get up and go," which they sometimes describe as "blue days." If you also notice a decreased sex drive, it is more likely to be low testosterone causing your low mood. Low testosterone levels can be caused by taking oral contraceptives, so be sure to ask your doctor to check your free testosterone level if you are on a birth control pill and experiencing more frequent blues and lower libido. Other possible hormonal causes include less than optimal thyroid hormone levels (particularly free T3) and reduced growth hormone secretion.

## DEPRESSION

*Q: I am forty-two years old, 245 pounds. I have next to no libido. Don't sleep with my husband. Have mood swings. I would love to lose the weight, but I can't. I know my hormones are totally out of whack and have been for years. I want to get well.*

DR. SEAN BREEN: The first step is to get blood work to check all your hormone levels, in addition to vitamin D and other nutrient levels. It is not uncommon for patients this age to have suboptimal thyroid levels, decreased levels of testosterone, vitamin D deficiency, and other nutrient deficiencies. Once your hormone levels are balanced the next step is to really study your diet. For example, patients who drink a lot of soda or diet soda get exposed to very high amounts of aspartame, which is an excitatory neurotransmitter that can cause psychiatric symptoms. Eating clean and drinking nothing but water for one month is a good start. Look at an elimination diet to see if there are foods that are contributing to the symptoms. Lastly, consider the environmental toxins that you may be harboring in fat cells. Things like heavy metal toxicity can cause a myriad of symptoms that typically get missed by the traditional medical doctor.

## FIBROIDS

*Q: Can you please tell me how to get rid of my uterine fibroids without surgery? I am forty-one. Is this hormone related?*

DR. PRUDENCE HALL: Uterine fibroids are benign growths on the uterus that are common to many women as they age. They are considered to be inflammatory in nature, like most benign and cancerous tumors are. They don't have to be removed unless they cause profuse, troublesome bleeding, bad cramping and pressure, or are rapidly growing in size. I love treating fibroids naturally and suggest the following: first eliminate any dietary foods that can cause inflammation. The main ones are gluten, dairy, soy, peanuts, sugar, eggs, and red meat. Next, drink a nice healthy green drink for breakfast, made of detoxifying greens such as kale, dandelion greens, celery, cilantro, or parsley, and also add turmeric and ginger. Shakes made from natural plant-based proteins are also helpful, and enzymes are important to seal the deal. These "rotor-rooters" go into the body to dissolve abnormal tissue. I love the PuraDyme enzymes, which I feel are the highest quality available. Take four to six of their digestive enzymes (LiyfZymes) with each meal, and then on an empty stomach take six to eight of the supersystemic enzymes called Puraliyf. You can follow your progress with pelvic ultrasounds. Good luck!

## POLYPS

*Q: I am forty-eight years old. I had a polyp removed last October. My next period, I bled twice as much as my regular periods; I thought I'd bleed to death. The doctor put me on a three-month course of birth control. I don't know what to do once the course of treatment is over. Not to mention no sex drive left. What solution(s) do you have to offer? Thanks.*

DR. THERESA RAMSEY: First of all, it is best to inform whoever removed the polyp about the heavy bleeding. He or she is the best one to evaluate whether this may be related to the procedure performed. Putting a woman on birth control, oftentimes continuous, is a common treatment for heavy bleeding. Although this helps the heavy bleeding, it does not address the underlying cause, which likely is related to your hormones. The uterine lining is stimulated by estrogen and clearly you have plenty of this as is evident from the monthly bleeding. Estrogen will cause the lining to thicken each month and part of this is what you slough. Progesterone has an important role of opposing the stimulating effects of estrogen. I refer to progesterone as the disciplinarian of estrogen. If there is plenty of estrogen around and not enough progesterone, there will be heavy bleeding, and this is common in a woman nearing menopause. Typically progesterone levels decline before estrogen levels do and heavy bleeding will result. In the end, what you need is progesterone and enough of it to oppose the effects of your estrogen. There are many options for starting prescribed progesterone, but you definitely want to make sure it is bioidentical (e.g., Prometrium or compounded progesterone) and not medroxy progesterone acetate (e.g., Provera). Starting progesterone will offer you more benefits than just controlling the bleeding. It protects your breasts and uterus from cancer and can help you sleep better, not to mention help abate hot flashes and night sweats. You will want to take enough to slow the bleeding.

Irregular bleeding may continue, though, and this is simply the nature of perimenopause, as your hormones go up and down differently than they did earlier in your life. As far as the sex drive goes, be sure to have your doctor test your free testosterone and DHEA-sulfate levels, as these are important hormones that tend to be low at this time in a woman's life, and get you started on a dose that is right for you.

## SALIVA TESTING AND
## BIRTH CONTROL PILLS

*Q: I understand that saliva hormone testing is not accurate if I'm taking birth control pills. How can it be accurately tested if I don't want to stop taking the pill? I find it keeps me on an even keel for at least the time being. I am fifty and don't have any problems (yet!).*

DR. JOSEPH RAFFAELE: As with many things, the truth is somewhere in the middle. Saliva testing is relatively accurate for testosterone and can be used when a woman is on birth control pills. However, birth control pills contain a very potent estrogen, called ethinyl estradiol, that takes over the menstrual cycle, rendering saliva testing for estradiol, estriol, *and* progesterone useless. (It would also be relatively pointless to check *blood* levels for estrogen and progesterone while a patient is on a birth control pill.) Birth control pills put you on an even keel, but they come with a price in adverse physiological changes. You also won't be able to tell when you have gone through menopause (or even if you've entered perimenopause) while you are on the pill.

## MEMORY FOG

*Q: I decided in the last year to have bioidentical creams made up by my compounding pharmacy. I have been on them for almost one year, and my memory still has not gotten back to normal. I still am in a fog all the time!*

DR. GOWRI ROCCO: You have definitely taken the right steps by starting BHRT creams. If you have been on the creams for a year now, you should have felt much improvement in your memory and brain fog. If not, I suggest getting your estradiol, progesterone, total/free and bioavailable testosterone, and DHEA levels retested. It is important you are not being undertreated and that these values are in optimal ranges for you. Testosterone, especially, is important not only for increased libido, but also for increased cognitive functioning. Other supplements that greatly help with memory recall and improving brain fog are phosphatidylserine, fish or krill oil, and vitamin $D_3$. It is important that you are not deficient in any of these levels as well. Phosphatidylserine is a brain nutrient that has been shown to improve memory, learning, and other cognitive functioning. It is easily tolerated. It is best to take 200 mg of it with 250 mg of DHA+EPA omega-3 fish oil or krill oil. Vitamin $D_3$ is best to keep at levels between 80 and 85 ng/mL. Generally, to keep $D_3$ at this level, it depends on the blood results, and may require between 5,000 and 10,000 IU daily. Work with your physician.

## RACING HEART

*Q: I have been having heart-racing episodes since I was forty-three years old . . . tests reveal nothing is wrong with my heart, yet it will race out of control during my sleep and sometimes when I'm awake. Why? When this happens while I'm asleep and I wake up to it beating out of control, I simply change positions and within a minute or so my heart rate goes back to normal. I can actually feel some type of "surge" going through my body when the episodes begin; is this from my hormones fluctuating and if so, what can I do to get things under control?*

DR. THERESA RAMSEY: It is common to have heart symptoms as our hormones change. There are two steps for you to take. One is to have a cardiac workup with a cardiologist for a stress echo and Holter monitor. The other is to have your entire hormone panel tested. Since you are cycling, the best time of the month to do your blood work is within the week before anticipated menses. Make sure you are having your blood work reviewed by a hormone specialist, because if a physician is not a hormone specialist, he or she will tell you that your levels "normally" drop as we age. A hormone specialist will tell you that although it is "normal," it is not "optimal." Hormone specialists understand how to optimize hormone levels, which brings with it symptom resolution as well as preventive aging.

## HOT FLASHES AND NIGHT SWEATS

*Q: I'm forty-nine and still have regular periods. However, I'm experiencing hot flashes and night sweats. As a result my doctor put me on estrogen for the hot flashes. Unfortunately, it made me swell and bloat. My breasts became painful, and the bleeding and cramps were intense, so I stopped the estrogen and felt better. However, now I have hot flashes and can't sleep at night. I'm damned if I do and damned if I don't.*

DR. NEIL ROUZIER: You are entering perimenopause, during which time your hormones will fluctuate from very high to very low. There are two ways to describe perimenopause: (1) *Anything that happens is normal.* This is due to the extreme fluctuations of hormones. (2) Perimenopause is also termed no-man's-land as no man knows how to treat it (as in your case) and no man wants to deal with it (maybe your husband). Let's review some physiology to understand why you have what you have and then we will understand how to fix it.

In the past, doctors treated perimenopausal women with birth control pills to wipe out ovarian function and thereby eliminate the yo-yoing effect of their hormones. Many women, however, do not want to take BCPs due to side effects and complications.

Normally in premenopause, your pituitary hormones (FSH) remain within the normal range of around 10 or less. As time goes on, however, the production of a particular hormone, inhibin, from the ovaries diminishes and the brain (pituitary gland) senses the loss of this hormone and tries to compensate for loss. The brain then releases follicle-stimulating hormone in an attempt to stimulate the ovaries to produce more inhibin. This increase in FSH increases production of all hormones from the ovaries, primarily estrogen. The less and less inhibin the ovaries produce, then the higher the production of FSH by the pituitary to stimulate the production of inhibin. It is the loss of inhibin that results in the early symptoms of hot flashes and night sweats. And it is the increase in estrogen production by the ovaries that results in your symptoms of excess estrogen in spite of the fact that you are experiencing hot flashes. If we tested your estrogen level during a hot flash (when you would normally think that it would be very low), it is actually quite high. Remember that it is the loss of inhibin that first triggers hot flashes in perimenopause. Your doctor interpreted that your hot flashes were due to loss of estrogen, when in reality your estrogen was quite high as evidenced by your symptoms of excess estrogen. In fact, your estrogen can be two to three times normal in perimenopause and the inhibin will fall to zero. When the inhibin falls to zero, inhibin no longer inhibits FSH; production of FSH increases, which increases production of estrogen to excess, which causes symptoms of excess estrogen in spite of continued hot flashes. See how important it is to understand the physiology behind perimenopause in order to understand how to treat it? And it's not with estrogen as many physicians think.

Since your ovaries are already working overtime to produce excess estrogen from increased production of FSH, you do not need estrogen at this time, which in fact will increase your symptoms of excess estrogen (breast swelling, bleeding, bloating).

The treatment is, therefore, to oppose the high levels of estrogen that you produce in perimenopause. The treatment is simply the same as for PMS and that is high-dose progesterone. The higher the estrogen, the greater the symptoms, the more progesterone is needed. Progesterone is excellent at alleviating the hot flashes and symptoms of perimenopause. It also opposes the side effects of increased estrogen. Oral progesterone is also soporific, which improves sleep and eliminates the insomnia of perimenopause. Progesterone is an excellent sleep aid and antianxiety treatment, in addition to being the treatment of choice for perimenopause.

Testosterone is also an important therapeutic hormone for hot flashes, loss of strength and energy at menopause, and for the loss of muscle and metabolism (and weight gain) seen at menopause. Even though you may not need estrogen at this time, optimizing all your other hormones (progesterone, testosterone, DHEA, thyroid) will help improve symptoms and well-being and will make your friends wonder how you skated through perimenopause so easily. There is also nothing better that you can do to maintain your optimal health.

## DIDN'T FIND RELIEF FROM REPLACEMENT

*Q: I have tried hormone replacement and did not see much relief. I was using the Vivelle patch and progesterone in pill form. I am now fifty-two and experiencing an increase in weight gain, hot flashes, and an overall feeling of worthlessness, tiredness, no libido, no desire for much of anything. . . . Should I try the hormones again?*

DR. RON ROTHENBERG: Optimizing hormones requires balancing all the hormones that are deficient to produce optimal results in quality of life. First, let's consider what you were taking. The patch you were using is bioidentical estradiol but does not contain the weak cancer-protective estrogen, E3 or estriol. "Biest" is a mixture of estradiol and estriol, which can be made by a compounding pharmacy and is preferred by most women. You state that you were taking a "progesterone pill." I hope that was bioidentical progesterone but sometimes "progestins" are referred to as progesterone by those who are not experienced in this field. (Please see my earlier explanation of the difference between the two in terms of cancer risks [page 180].) There is also a major difference in terms of quality of life. Bioidentical progesterone is a natural mood stabilizer and brain builder, and it helps to produce natural sleep. It can be a natural diuretic and can help with weight loss. Progestins, or artificial nonbioidentical progesterone, often have the opposite effect. The use of the "patch" and the progesterone pill are to treat estrogen and progesterone deficiency; however, the third hormone that is often missed by traditional practitioners is testosterone. In replacing the estrogen and progesterone alone, your available testosterone level drops, which for most women will decrease your libido, decrease your motivation, increase fat, and generally give you an off-balance feeling. I would definitely consider restarting hormone replacement, but in doing so, check all your hormones. Look at thyroid and cortisol, testosterone, and insulin, and be sure all deficiencies are being addressed. In addition, each woman is unique and her balance of hormones is unique. One size does not fit all and the balance of hormones must be optimized for you.

## CANDIDA AND YEAST

*Q: Have you ever discussed the impact candida has on hormone absorption? It blocks the cells from receiving the bioidentical hormones. After we discovered this, I went on the diet suggested by the Hotze Clinic in Houston and it changed my life.*

DR. RON ROTHENBERG: Maintaining a balance of hormones does require maintaining balance in your body. Gut health, which includes candida and other dysbioses or overgrowth infections, triggers inflammation. Elevated cortisol can increase blood sugar and this can increase your tendency for candida overgrowth. Inflammation can have negative impacts on health from head to toe. It is important to look for food sensitivities as well. Treatment of this imbalance is primarily dietary with a reduction of high carbohydrates, but also would include omega-3 fish oil, probiotics, possibly digestive enzymes, and stress reduction.

Bioidentical hormone treatment should always be done in the setting of optimizing lifestyle and wellness so it should include nutrition, exercise, stress reduction, and eliminating toxicities and underlying infections.

*Q: I have candida. Talk about disrupting every system in the body. Are there natural herbal products out there that you could recommend instead of drugs that make it worse?*

DR. RACHEL BURNETT: Many people suffer from yeast overgrowth and it is commonly overlooked. It is important to note that yeast is a normal organism, but given the opportunity (and there are many in our modern-day culture) it can easily overgrow and manifest as symptoms that are very troublesome. The first step would be to get tested, since some of the symptoms of yeast overgrowth such as bloating and fatigue can be due to other causes. Treating presumptively only to find out later that yeast was really not the underlying cause can prolong recovery and result in unnecessary spending. I recommend doing a stool test that uses advanced-technology DNA analysis that is very sensitive. Most functional laboratories offer these tests that your doctor can order for you. Another benefit of using a test like this is that it has the ability to test not only which pharmaceuticals the condition may be sensitive or resistant to, but also which botanical medicine would work. Having tested hundreds of patients, I have found that my patients have the most success with a pharmaceutical-grade caprylic acid or grapefruit seed extract. It is important to note that killing the yeast is the easiest part. Preventing its regrowth is the challenge. That is where a good discussion with your doctor comes in, so you can really look at contributing factors. Oftentimes there are dietary considerations; sometimes it involves a close look at other obstacles and how to avoid them. The upside is that you will learn how yeast overgrowth manifests in you and then if it returns you will know why it came back and how to kill it.

## WEIGHT GAIN

*Q: My doctor told me that, because I am overweight, he cannot accurately determine my hormone levels. He says that my estrogen levels are high because I am fat. How can I know if or when I might need to address hormone deficiencies, and how do I go about it?*

DR. GAIL GAGNON: Being overweight does not prevent you from having your hormones levels tested. You can measure your estrogen level (as well as progesterone, testosterone, cortisol, and thyroid levels) via blood, urine, or saliva. If your menstrual cycle is regular (every month), the best time to measure your hormones is on day 19, 20, or 21 of your cycle. During these days your hormones should be at their highest levels. If you are deficient, then you are a candidate for hormone replacement therapy. Your excess weight could be due to insulin resistance related to estrogen, progesterone, testosterone, thyroid, and/or cortisol imbalance. All of these hormones can be measured and replaced, as needed, with bioidentical hormones leading to increased energy and decreased food cravings, and making it easier to implement a healthy weight loss program. I recommend you find a bioidentical hormone physician, have your hormone levels tested, and, if needed, implement bioidentical hormone replacement therapy.

*Q: I just saw an Internet commercial for hormone weight loss. It said that leptin is the trigger for keeping us heavy. What are your thoughts?*

DR. PRUDENCE HALL: Weight loss is an important topic for most of us, because during perimenopause and menopause it is common to put on thirty pounds or more, sometimes without even changing our eating or exercise habits. The weight gain is often due to fluctuating and low levels of estrogens, which trigger anxiety eating and inefficient digestion, and decreases in neuro-transmitters in the brain, which stimulate depression and hunger. This is the time many food intolerances/allergies develop, because in perimenopause and menopause, we lose our digestive enzymes and acids. This creates inflammation in the body, which packs on the pounds. Leptin and ghrelin also play roles in appetite control and hunger, but more important, our thyroid function frequently declines dramatically in perimenopause, and low thyroid hormones add lots of weight. Increased stress also does, and the female body definitely feels stressed as it experiences a decline in estradiol levels.

*Q: I've been trying to figure out if the weight around my middle, fatigue, and horrible constipation (around my period) is caused by perimenopause. When I look at symptoms of perimenopause, none of my symptoms show up, and I'm not experiencing the symptoms that are listed. What is happening?*

DR. EVELYN BRUST: The symptoms of weight gain around the middle, constipation, and fatigue may be caused by any number of different conditions. My recommendation for you would be to work with a physician who is an expert in metabolic and hormone balance.

A thorough multifactorial workup might be indicated in your case so as not to miss anything, and to determine the best personalized treatment plan for you. Working with an expert may help you figure out how to be the healthiest you can be.

## HYSTERECTOMY

*Q: Tell me about BHRT after a hysterectomy.*

DR. RACHEL BURNETT: Oftentimes, when a woman is close to menopause and if there is any abnormal bleeding or complaint related to her uterus, she is told that her best option is to get a full hysterectomy (i.e., hormone-making ovaries out, too) because, as they may tell her, her ovaries will stop working soon anyway and she will minimize her risk of uterine or ovarian cancer if she gets them out. Trusting her doctors, she goes down this path only to learn quickly that a life without hormones or with estrogen only, if her doctor puts her on any hormones, is a very different life than she imagined.

The idea here is that the estrogen may manage any hot flashes she experiences and this estrogen replacement will be at the lowest dose possible to manage the symptoms for the shortest amount of time. Libido plummets, depression starts to set in, weight gain appears, and sleep disappears. Moreover, the risk for heart disease, cognitive decline, osteoporosis, diabetes, macular degeneration, among other chronic diseases, just went through the roof. A comprehensive look at one's hormones is critical at this point and the sooner bioidentical hormone replacement is started, the more benefit there will be in the long run. The key tests are estradiol, progesterone, free testosterone, and DHEA-sulfate. Oftentimes thyroid (Free T3 in particular), although not an ovarian hormone, is not optimized and we will look at this also since a well-functioning thyroid helps us feel our best. Once a woman starts hormones, it is important that there is good follow-up with her doctor to make sure the levels are enough not only to make her feel better, but also to protect her from chronic disease. Many doctors do not follow up and simply give prescriptions and let women go on their way. Bioidentical hormone replacement therapy is individualized and often fine-tuned after considering laboratory results together with how the woman feels.

*Q: How are hormones correctly tested after a hysterectomy?*

DR. SEAN BREEN: The most accurate way to test hormone levels following a hysterectomy is through simple blood work. The specific hormones that you should have checked are progesterone, estradiol, testosterone (free and total), follicle-stimulating hormone (FSH), luteinizing hormone (LH), IGF-1 (growth hormone production), and DHEA-sulphate. If you had your ovaries removed, then you will need bioidentical hormones. If they left your ovaries in, then you just need to make sure that you are still producing enough estradiol, testosterone, and progesterone. It is quite common for hormone levels to decline slightly as a result of having the uterus removed because of mild loss of secondary blood vessels to the ovaries.

# THE WRAP-UP

I love this letter from one of my readers. It makes me smile. . . .

I gave up my singing career because I was afraid of everything, afraid of what people thought of me, afraid of forgetting the lyrics (and I usually did), and of just not having the nerves to step out into the world. I quit singing for eight years and then in getting my hormones balanced, I started to feel like maybe I could sing in public again! I gained confidence, stepped out, and learned to love myself. Three years later I now have my own CD and a career that I love.

—Cat C.

Isn't it wonderful to hear a woman singing the praises of her next transition? That she found the answer, and now perimenopause is a breeze *and* she's "singing" again?

Now it's time for YOU! It's time too for you to find your song, *sing it,* and be fully alive. To be "of" life rather than "out of" life's energy.

> You are entering the most exciting phase of your life.

The angst is over; you now have a much better idea of who you are, and the gift of your wisdom is beginning to shine. You also have the gift of perspective. You can look back and remember when you felt like a walking ball of confusion and insecurities. Now is YOUR time to be a grown woman at her best.

We do get better with age, but up until now women have bought into the advertising that says we are "less than" as we get older. Not true! I'm sitting on top of that wisdom/perspective mountain right now and I *love* the view! I'm able to see so clearly. It makes each day light, bright, happy, and upbeat. But if I were not hormonally balanced, I would be hanging on to life by my fingernails.

I chose to take charge of my health; I feel good, I'm healthy, and I'm cutting-edge by taking control of my body and my quality of life. I am the contractor of my body. I hire qualified doctors to be my subcontractors. It's the new way to go to the doctor; *you* are the one in charge. And you can be because you have now armed yourself with knowledge. *You* can ask the intelligent questions. *You* have information that allows you to have critical thinking, figuring out the puzzle of your own chemistry with the help of your doctor. It's your body. No one is ever going to care about it as much as you, so taking charge and care of it should be a no-brainer.

I am happy and proud to bring information that can help you along during this difficult passage. I hope I have made it clear and broken it down, so that it is simple and easy to embrace. I've tried to give you the answers to the questions that so many readers have asked, so as to give you the tools to live a drug-free, healthy, sexy, happy life.

At present, our medical schools are teaching fifty-year-old medicine. Every answer to every disease and condition has a pill attached to it. If you look around at our senior generation, you see for yourselves that they are not doing very well on all the pills they have been given over the years. It's a cruel hoax; they trusted and they believed that medicine knew best.

We get confused because we have been raised to believe doctors are supposed to know everything. That's a lot of pressure for your doctor. Stay with your doctor for the things he or she knows, but go to the right doctor if you are looking for hormone balance (someone who specializes in BHRT).

Doctors are good people we hire to take care of our bodies. But they are not *in charge* of our bodies . . . that is your responsibility. You must feed it right, sleep it properly, think good thoughts, and do your research to understand the language of your body and not allow any part of it to deteriorate. Your brain is a big part of this management. With all the chemicals and toxins abundant in our environment, maintaining health is more difficult today than at any time in the history of humanity.

As I've discussed an entire generation before us is lost in a sea of pills. Just when our planet needs wisdom more than ever to deal with the chaos we can't seem to escape, we desperately need "the elders of the tribe" in order to access their perspective, but sadly we have so few to go to. Our wisdom pool has been wiped out by bad choices, environmental challenges, and allopathic medicine's overreliance on a pill for every pain. Foggy brains, an inability to think or reason, rampant Alzheimer's—all are tragic. Don't let this be you.

When my book *The Sexy Years* came out in 2004, no one had ever heard of bioidentical hormones. I was attacked on TV and in print for suggesting there was a better way. But the information resonated with women readers and they started thinking for themselves. As a result, the sales of Wyeth Pharmaceutical's main hormone drugs dropped by 72 percent. I can't say for sure it was my book that started the change, but I'm sure my message had impact. No wonder I was being attacked. If my theory was true, it would affect their bottom line. Regardless, many thousands of women went to their doctors and began their regimens of BHRT. And they got better.

Women came up to me on the street and cried; they said that their lives had been saved. Yet a lot of women were still white-knuckling needlessly each day, and instead taking a coterie of pills.

Your generation has a better chance. We are right ahead of you and you can look to those of us who chose to go another way to see how well we are doing. I want you to want what I have. The good news is that now you know how to get it.

At this very moment we are all being bombarded by toxins and stresses. Our food is not as nutritious as it used to be, and now it's more important than ever to recognize the weaknesses of our modern lifestyle and do what we can to fill in the gaps. Our bodies need real food, real exercise, and real respect. The air we breathe, the water we drink, and the food we eat will determine our health and outlook. As hormones decline these choices are more important than ever.

Your body needs and requires tender loving care and the more you understand the effects of making good choices relative to diet and lifestyle, the more likely you will experience enjoyable aging and smooth hormonal transitions. Paying attention to your strengths and weaknesses—what makes you sick and what makes you well—will empower you to make positive choices. As Dr. Hall says in the foreword, "Choices do matter."

You are the hope for the future health of your children. That you are making corrections in your chemical makeup in peri-menopause is going to give you a quality of life that will not include unnecessary suffering and terrible symptoms of meno-pause. As you age, your dosages will change and increase accord-ing to your symptoms. You will get good at this because no one knows your body better than you. If you begin now and get your-self well and balanced, you (and hopefully your generation) will have a real shot at healthy, vibrant longevity.

You will maintain your wisdom, and with each passing year as you feel better and better, you will not be a drain on society; you will be an asset, a *productive* member of the tribe.

You can no longer look to your grandparents. Nothing about our planet is the same as the one they were born into fifty or more years ago. Toxins didn't exist to the extent they do today, and stress was not nearly as prevalent as it is today. Today's world accelerates aging and blunts hormone production in the process.

The message in this book is not to go to the doctor as a child anymore. Empower yourself with information about how your body works; it will allow you to discuss your health intelligently with your doctor. Together you can decide on a personalized plan for your ongoing health. It's up to you to choose optimal health. Remember, you hire your doctor! *You* are the contractor. As you continue to age you will hire other doctors specializing in new medicine to manage and maintain all your other parts. Peri-menopause is a passage . . . a passage into the next phase of your life called menopause.

I will tell you again. I have nothing but glowing remarks to be made about my aging experience. I feel I have my "edge," and I feel relevant and sexy. It's a great feeling. Replacing my hormones is the most important thing I have ever done for my health and well-being.

I know in perimenopause you feel too young for what is hap-pening to your body, but you have been born into a new world. The doctors I recommend understand this. They are not "stuck" in the old medicine. In fact, I attend doctors' conferences regu-larly to learn and upgrade my information. And when I am at-tending meetings like A4M (American Academy of Anti-Aging Medicine) or ACAM (American College for Advancement in

Medicine), I am thoroughly impressed by the enthusiasm these new doctors have for their work. They share information with one another gratefully, and in doing so, we all benefit.

You can make this passage an entry into a better phase of life. With proper replacement, nutrition, sleep, stress reduction, and supplementation you will look and feel great. Your husband or partner will be turned on by your vitality, great health, and sexiness. And you will carry with you an air of confidence reserved only for those of us who have figured out how to do this right.

Go for it. Take charge of your life and be the one to determine your outcome. Enjoy perimenopause!

# RESOURCES

The book isn't truly over . . . so don't skip these valuable pieces!

The rest of the book includes some very important tools to keep in your back pocket to help you enjoy a smooth ride through this transition.

They include the following:

- The Symptom Solver
- Finding a Doctor
- Getting Tested
- Letters from Women Like You
- Further Reading

# THE SYMPTOM SOLVER

When a woman is hormonally imbalanced, the body ceases to operate at its peak and suffers a slow and insidious decline. That's why it's important to test your hormone levels so that your health adviser can connect the dots and determine if these symptoms are perimenopausal. It's difficult to describe the enormous relief women feel when they balance their hormones. Most women come up to me and cry because it has so changed their lives.

I asked my friend Bill Faloon at Life Extension to offer suggestions and solutions for how to stop a symptom in its tracks, while your body does its healing.

## BREAKTHROUGH BLEEDING

Sadly, I learned the hard way. My uterus was taken out surgically (a decision I regret) to remove the "evidence" of bleeding. I say evidence because it removed the symptom, but it did not deal with the *reason* why I was bleeding. I had started bleeding to the point I would hemorrhage. One day my husband walked into the bathroom to find me on the floor passed out in a pool of blood. We thought there was nothing that could be done but to remove my uterus.

My sister was experiencing the same thing, and after a couple of trips to the emergency room, she was also scheduled to have her uterus removed. It was around that time I learned of "rhythmic" cycling and I told my sister she should try taking her hormones in a rhythm before she did something as drastic as having a hysterectomy. Within a couple of months of using this method, her periods normalized, the bleeding stopped, and she was able to save this valuable body part.

Those of us who were at the forefront of taking bioidentical hormones were at the mercy of the few doctors with the courage to prescribe them. Due to the lack of a complete picture at that time, the importance of finding the right dosage for each woman was not understood. They felt that giving the smallest amount was safest, but I and many other women were *underdosed*. We felt better, but we weren't getting enough to do the job; we were still imbalanced. I require large dosages of all the hormones. So for me, fifteen years ago, low-dose estrogen and two weeks of low-dose progesterone caused me to lose my uterus even though I was cycling. That is why I began bleeding.

I believe that had I been able to take larger doses of progesterone in a cyclic fashion while taking my hormones I would have been able to save my uterus.

## Solutions for Breakthrough Bleeding

Have your blood tested for estrogens (estradiol and estrone), progesterone, DHEA, thyroid, and testosterone. You'll get your results back in a few days and be able to talk to a health adviser about simple lifestyle changes or seeing a doctor who will prescribe the optimal dose of bioidentical hormones based on your blood test results.

## Safety Caveat

Although hormonal fluctuation is a common cause of break-through bleeding during perimenopause, there are other potential causes such as infections (e.g., in the uterus), hypothyroidism, medications (e.g., anticoagulants), stress, a significant change in body weight (weight gain or loss), internal polyps/fibroids/ovarian masses, and most worrisome, gynecological cancers. Make sure you report any chronic, abnormal bleeding problems to your gynecologist.

# CHOCOLATE AND FOOD CRAVINGS

You don't want to do it, but there you are; it's late and you are craving . . . what . . . then you spy chocolate! Any kind, you don't care; it's interesting that when you are having cravings, it doesn't have to be good-quality Belgian chocolate, any chocolate—even baking chocolate—will do just fine. What is that about?

It's your hormones again. When progesterone levels aren't sufficient to balance estrogen, your body attempts to "fix" things by producing more progesterone. Magnesium is required to produce progesterone and chocolate is high in magnesium. The body in its wisdom is triggering this craving so you can get this very important mineral.

However, chocolate is also high in theobromine, a substance that artificially and dangerously overstimulates your adrenals. If your adrenals aren't functioning optimally your body craves this "hit," but too much chocolate, and in turn theobromine, can cause adrenal fatigue, which can lead to hypoglycemia or low blood sugar. Now you've got an insulin problem and as a result you will start craving sugars and carbohydrates. Now the chain reaction has begun: the excess carbs and sugars trigger the release of excess insulin, which leads to low blood sugar and adrenal crash requiring another hit of sugar or carbs, and your body is now in motion for weight gain.

### Solutions for Chocolate Cravings

In addition to having your hormones tested (as all women experiencing perimenopausal symptoms should do), have your blood levels of glucose and insulin checked. To control excess insulin levels that can cause cravings for chocolate and sugar, take the following before most meals:

Coffee Genic Green Coffee Bean Extract, 350–400 mg
Glycemic Transglucosidase, 225 mg
LuralLean, 2,000 mg

Take three capsules NeuroMag (magnesium L-threonate) each day.

The health benefits of magnesium are enormous, and magnesium L-threonate specifically targets the brain and nervous system. It may help you cut back on chocolate cravings.

If snacking is a problem, you can try taking one capsule of Optimized Saffron twice a day. Saffron has been shown in clinical studies to target emotional factors involved in food cravings. (For more information on easy weight loss, go to SexyForever.com.)

# CONSTIPATION

Constipation now affects approximately 27 percent of the population of Western countries. There are 2.5 million visits to the doctor and 92,000 hospitalizations a year involving constipation. Laxative sales exceed several hundred million dollars a year.

Not surprisingly, constipation is an offshoot of a toxic gut; the more severe the toxicity, the worse the problem. I have letters from readers (women in their thirties) telling me they only have one bowel movement every three weeks! This is a serious body dysfunction. A healthy person has one to three bowel movements a DAY!

Toxins accumulate when you are constipated; in fact, the purpose of a daily bowel movement is to rid the body of toxins. Toxins may interfere with communication between the brain and the thyroid, eventually leading to low thyroid function, which can cause constipation, fatigue, and exhaustion (exhaustipation).

The buildup of toxins in the brain may also contribute to depression. What do we do when we are depressed? We look for anything to take the pain away, and that is usually alcohol and/or opiates.

Opiate-induced constipation downgrades the immune system, creating severe intestinal permeability or what is known as "leaky gut" syndrome. Leaky gut is where the inflammation and toxins "eat" little holes in the lining of your intestine, ostensibly allowing toxins to "leak out" into your bloodstream.

If these toxins are not cleared out of the body, you can remain in a state of inflammation and will most likely resort to pain medications and laxatives to alleviate your suffering. There are many factors contributing to constipation: dehydration, lack of fiber, lack of beneficial bacteria, lack of B vitamins, certain medications, chronic stress, and hormonal imbalance. Another significant contributor to constipation is *insufficient peristalsis*. The term *peristalsis* refers to a series of organized muscle contractions that moves food through the digestive tract. Insufficient peristalsis means there is not enough colonic contractile activity to completely evacuate one's bowels.

Constipation, as most people know, is sometimes caused by

a lack of fiber in the diet. Fast food, poor quality oils, and excess sugar all take their toll on your ability to have normal bowel movements, but the biggest culprit compromising your ability to have a normal functioning system is hormonal in origin and that culprit is low thyroid. Hormones regulate every system in your body, which may present the answer to what may be a chronic, debilitating, and ultimately very unhealthy problem.

## Solutions for Chronic Constipation

There are a number of synthetic and natural products that produce a "colon cleaning" effect, but they often contain questionable ingredients. For example, *polyethylene glycol* (PEG) is used in both industrial manufacturing and medicine. You can find it on the shelves of most pharmacies without the need for a prescription. The question for those with unrelenting constipation is would you rather ingest an ingredient (PEG) used in detergents and organic solvents, or nutrients you may already be taking in tablet or capsule form for their health benefits? (The medical establishment prefers you take PEG.)

You don't have to experiment with these types of artificial laxatives. By taking nutritional powder mixes containing vitamin C with magnesium and/or potassium on an empty stomach, you're likely to see results within an hour or two.

For example, one or more teaspoons of buffered, effervescent *magnesium ascorbate crystals* will evacuate the bowel within thirty to ninety minutes if taken on an empty stomach with several glasses of water. This powdered formula provides 3,000 mg of vitamin C and 170 mg of magnesium in each teaspoon. The dose of these effervescent crystals needs to be individually adjusted so it will not cause diarrhea.

The suggested number of times these nutritional colon cleanses can be used is about three times a week.

Those with kidney impairment should use caution when taking high doses of magnesium or potassium as your kidneys may not be able to handle them. Congestive heart failure patients may also have problems excreting large doses of magnesium and potassium through their kidneys. Those who suffer irritable bowel syndrome of the diarrhea-predominate type should avoid these formulas as it will likely worsen their problem.

It is important to drink lots of water after taking these powdered nutrient mixes as they will draw water from surrounding tissues into the colon to facilitate passage of feces. By increasing the volume of water in the intestine, stools are softened, intestinal muscle contraction is stimulated, and bowel evacuation is prompted.

Until an individual dose is ascertained by trial and error, these nutrient powders may create temporary diarrhea. Those with chronic constipation can learn how to dose their powdered nutrients to achieve optimal individual relief.

To improve intestinal health:

- Make sure to have your blood tested for thyroid hormone. If thyroid is low, ask your doctor to prescribe the proper dose of Armour or Cytomel to restore your thyroid status.
- On a daily basis, take 30 to 80 billion culture count probiotic, twice daily, to restore bacterial balance and pH of the colon. The colon contains a robust population of beneficial bacteria that help digest remaining nutrients. Beneficial bacteria include *Lactobacillus acidophilus* and *Bifidobacterium bifidum* (*B. bifidum*). Maintaining a healthy population of these beneficial bacteria is essential for proper digestion. Several recent studies demonstrate significant improvements in measures of gastrointestinal well-being, decreases in digestive symptoms such as gas and bloating, and increases in health-related quality of life during bifidobacteria supplementation.

- Consider fiber in capsule form or eat three cups of fibrous vegetables. Not all constipated people benefit from fiber, especially those suffering from *insufficient peristalsis*. These individuals usually need a colon cleanse three times a week to fully evacuate their bowels.

- Take digestive enzymes, one or two capsules with each meal, to help digest food and absorb nutrients.

- To stimulate peristalsis, take several teaspoons of effervescent magnesium ascorbate crystals with several glasses of water on an empty stomach; you're likely to see immediate results within an hour or two. Consuming this nutritional colon cleanse three times weekly provides significant constipation relief for many people.

## ENDOMETRIOSIS

Endometriosis is another very painful affliction that plagues many perimenopausal women. The symptoms are cramping and abdominal pain resulting from the cells of endometrial (uterine) tissue that somehow migrate outside the uterus. They can be scattered anywhere throughout the pelvic area, attaching to the ovaries, the bladder wall, as well as the intestinal walls and membranes in the abdomen. The endometrial tissue responds to the monthly surges of estrogen by becoming blood filled, and at menstruation when the uterine endometrium is shed, the endometrial cells also "shed" blood. But this blood has nowhere to go. The blood in the tissues creates local inflammation, which is very painful in the pelvic and abdominal tissues. Endometriosis is aggravated by estrogen dominance and birth control pills.

Endometriosis disappears during pregnancy only to flare up again after delivery, so this suggests that the sex hormones are involved and that the high progesterone levels of pregnancy may be the important factor.

Dr. John Lee, the first doctor to treat perimenopausal women with progesterone, is known to have successfully treated endometriosis in women by using high doses of progesterone cream to create a pseudopregnancy state from day 5 to day 28 of the cycle. This will most likely cause the pain to subside, but it can take three to four months.

## Solutions for Endometriosis

Natural progesterone is structurally identical to progesterone produced in the body and has been shown to reduce inflammation in endometriosis and limit the growth of uterine tissue.

Several other natural interventions may provide relief from symptoms of endometriosis.

- DHA and EPA are omega-3 fatty acids found in fish oil that help fight inflammation, which is a factor in endometriosis.
- Silymarin, an active component of milk thistle, has been shown to inhibit an inflammatory molecule that is commonly elevated in women with endometriosis. Additionally, components in milk thistle have demonstrated potent antioxidant and free-radical-scavenging activity.
- GLA is a beneficial omega-6 fatty acid found in borage seed oil that can reduce inflammation in the body by inhibiting the production of pro-inflammatory molecules commonly associated with endometriosis.
- Modulating the metabolism of estrogen is a strategy that may be helpful with endometriosis. I3C (indole-3-carbinol), found in cruciferous vegetables, may help increase the amount of weaker estrogens and decrease the amount of

stronger estrogens that are associated with cancer. Additionally, DIM, a metabolite of I3C, has been shown to have cancer-fighting effects.

- Calcium D-glucarate has been shown to inhibit an enzyme that is produced by bacteria in the gut that impairs the body's ability to adequately eliminate estrogen processed by the liver. Maintaining a higher ratio of weak estrogens to strong estrogens is important in promoting hormonal balance in endometriosis.

| Dosage Suggestions for Endometriosis | | |
|---|---|---|
| **NUTRIENT OR INTERVENTION** | **TYPICAL DAILY DOSE** | **SUGGESTED PRODUCTS** |
| Natural progesterone cream | Based on blood test results, symptoms, and physician prescribing directions. | Available over the counter or by prescription |
| Fish oil | 1,400 mg EPA and 1,000 mg DHA | Super Omega-3 EPA/DHA with Sesame Lignans and Olive Fruit Extract |
| Milk thistle extract | 1,500 mg standardized to 80% silymarin and 30% silibinins | Certified European Milk Thistle |
| Gamma-linolenic acid (GLA) | 300–600 mg | Mega GLA with Sesame Lignans |
| Indole-3-carbinol (I3C) 3,3'-diindolylmethane (DIM) | 80–160 mg  14–28 mg | Triple Action Cruciferous Vegetable Extract |
| Calcium D-glucarate | 200 mg | Calcium D-Glucarate |

# FIBROCYSTIC BREASTS

One sign of low iodine is fibrocystic breasts. Dr. Jonathan Wright claims that "if you take the right amount of iodine your fibrocystic disease will go away no matter how bad it is, and it works every time. (Very few things in medicine or anywhere else work every time, but this one does.) You don't need to take estriol, either, if you take enough iodine your body will make enough estriol for you." (To refresh, estriol is the safer component of a woman's estrogens.)Iodine deficiency interferes with optimum breast health, and intake of levels far higher than the recommended dietary allowance of 150 mcg may be required to achieve benefits.

You can test for iodine deficiency by dabbing a bit of iodine on your stomach. If it disappears in less than twenty-four hours you are iodine deficient. The faster it disappears the greater your deficiency.

### Solutions to Fibrocystic Breast Disease

In addition, women with fibrocystic breast disease may have abnormal ratios of omega-3 fatty acids. Improving the ratio of omega-3s to omega-6s can help reduce the inflammation associated with fibrocystic breasts.

- Gamma-linolenic acid (GLA) is a beneficial plant-derived omega-6 fatty acid that can play an important role in modulating inflammation throughout the body, especially when it is incorporated in the cells of the immune system. Additionally, GLA can supply the body with vital biochemical precursors with powerful anti-inflammatory effects.
- Research has shown that vitamin E can correct abnormal estrogen-progesterone ratios in some patients with abnormal cellular changes in their breasts.

- According to some alternative-care practitioners, a malfunctioning thyroid gland may worsen fibrocystic breast disease. An early study of 19 women with breast pain and nodularity caused by fibrocystic breast disease reported that almost half (47 percent) of the women had total relief after daily treatment with 0.1 mg of levothyroxine (Synthroid). Also, a study on thyroid hormones and fibrocystic breast disease showed that thyroid hormone levels were significantly lower in women with fibrocystic breast disease than in controls and it was concluded that there seemed to be a connection between disease occurrence and thyroid function. Taking daily iodine sourced from kelp and dulse can help support a healthy thyroid.
- Indole-3-carbinol (I3C) is a naturally occurring dietary compound found in cruciferous vegetables such as broccoli, cauliflower, Brussels sprouts, and cabbage. I3C's ability to break down estrogen into harmless forms rather than those linked to breast cancer, fight free radicals, and interfere with tumor cell reproduction makes it a useful therapy for fibrocystic breasts.

| Dosage Suggestions for Fibrocystic Breasts | | |
|---|---|---|
| NUTRIENT OR INTERVENTION | TYPICAL DAILY DOSE | SUGGESTED PRODUCTS |
| Iodine | 1,000–6,000 mcg | Sea-Iodine |
| Fish oil | 1,400 mg EPA and 1,000 mg DHA | Super Omega-3 EPA/DHA with Sesame Lignans and Olive Fruit Extract |
| Gamma tocopherol vitamin E (natural tocopherols mixed with sesame lignans) | 359 mg | Gamma E Tocopherol with Sesame Lignans |

| Gamma-linolenic acid (GLA) | 300–1,200 mg | Mega GLA with Sesame Lignans |
|---|---|---|
| Indole-3-carbinol (I3C) | 80–160 mg | Triple Action Cruciferous Vegetable Extract |
| High-potency, comprehensive multivitamin | One tablet twice daily | Two-Per-Day Tablets or Capsules |

# HEADACHE

Headaches have never been one of my overwhelming hormonal symptoms. I've had them of course but was never plagued and debilitated like so many women. I find my female friends with the worst GI problems—bloating and cramps—have the most headaches. This is not scientific, just something I've noticed. So getting your gut healthy could be an answer for you. If you find that you are suffering from more frequent headaches now, like so many women do at this time, here are some natural ways to treat them.

### Solutions for Chronic Headaches

- People who suffer from frequent headaches often have low levels of magnesium. Supplementing with magnesium may help headaches. If you experience diarrhea, take less.
- Dr. Prudence Hall, my gynecologist, suggests that a woman with migraines rub estrogen cream right on the temples to get it close to the brain. Many women have written me telling me this was the answer; that within a short period of time, the headache dissipated and they could get back to their lives. What I like about this approach is that no 'over-the-counter' drugs were needed. Chronic use of

over-the-counter (OTC) drugs like acetaminophen and ibu-
profen have lethal side effects. Do not use them to chronically treat headaches.

- Coffee and ice packs are also helpful as both caffeine and
ice cause blood vessels to constrict.

- Butterbur root extracts have properties that can reduce inflammation and dilate the blood vessels which can be very
helpful for headaches.

- Coenzyme $Q_{10}$ ($CoQ_{10}$) is an important antioxidant that
is quickly depleted in the brain due to its high energy de-
mands. Supplementing with it daily has been shown to be
helpful in preventing and reducing the frequency of headaches.

- Melatonin is a natural compound produced by the pineal
gland that helps regulate the sleep-wake cycle (i.e., circa-
dian rhythms), and has been clinically shown to possess
analgesic properties. Since melatonin is often found in
lower-than-normal levels among those who suffer frequent
headaches (especially during an attack), it is thought that
it may play an important role in headache cessation. Some
researchers hypothesize that headaches are triggered by an
irregularity in pineal gland function. When this imbalance
is corrected through melatonin supplementation, some patients experience an improvement in symptoms.

- The amino acid L-tryptophan is a precursor to serotonin.
Several lines of evidence indicate that low serotonin signal-
ing within the brain may precipitate headaches. Therefore,
supporting serotonin synthesis by providing precursors
like L-tryptophan may help avoid physiological conditions
that promote headaches.

| Dosage Suggestions for Chronic Headache | | |
|---|---|---|
| **NUTRIENT OR INTERVENTION** | **TYPICAL DAILY DOSE** | **SUGGESTED PRODUCTS** |
| Magnesium | 140 mg as magnesium L-threonate; 320 mg daily as magnesium citrate (the magnesium citrate may be repeated later in the day) | Neuro-Mag Magnesium L-Threonate; Magnesium Citrate |
| Natural progesterone cream | Based on blood test results, symptoms, and physician prescribing | Available by prescription or over the counter |
| Butterbur root | Standardized extract of 150 mg | Butterbur Extract with Standardized Rosmarinic Acid |
| Coenzyme $Q_{10}$ ($CoQ_{10}$), as ubiquinol | 100–300 mg | Super Ubiquinol $CoQ_{10}$ with Enhanced Mitochondrial Support |
| Melatonin | 0.3–5 mg before bed (sometimes up to 10 mg) | Melatonin |
| L-tryptophan | 500–2,000 mg | Optimized Tryptophan |

# HOT FLASHES

You know what these are if you've ever had one, but what to do to get you out of your misery? The remedy for hot flashes is bioidentical estrogen. Research shows that 97 percent of the symptoms of hot flashes are resolved by estrogen replacement.

But for some women estrogen alone is not sufficient. Low testosterone symptoms could be the culprit. Are you experiencing dry skin, a lack of interest in sex, a lack of progress in weight training? Testosterone helps generate estrogen in the brain where it needs to be to cure hot flashes. Resolving these issues often does the trick.

## Solutions for Hot Flashes

- Black cohosh may be effective for the treatment of hot flashes, mood disturbances, excessive sweating, palpitations, and vaginal dryness, but not all studies demonstrate efficacy.

- Daily treatment with the phytoestrogen genistein has been shown to safely decrease hot flashes up to 30 percent, but not all studies demonstrate efficacy. Again, low sex hormone status is the prime suspect for why it may not work in some.

- An extract of hops has been found to contain a previously unknown class of nonsteroidal phytoestrogens (*prenylflavonoids*), of which 8-prenylnaringenin (8-PN) is the most potent. In fact, clinical research has shown that most menopausal women who take it experience a rapid and significant reduction in hot flashes and other benefits.

- HMR lignan (containing 7-hydroxymatairesinol) a specific plant compound from the Norway Spruce can provide hot flash relief. A study indicated that postmenopausal women using HMR lignan daily over eight weeks experienced a 53.5 percent reduction in hot flashes as well as a reduction in other common menopausal complaints. In addition, clinical data suggest a lignan-rich diet supports breast health.

- The combination of testosterone and estrogen has been shown to reduce hot flashes, sleep disturbances, night sweats, and vaginal dryness. The use of estriol has also been shown to eliminate hot flashes and reduce night sweats in menopausal women. Nutrients can help, but proper hormone replacement is often essential.

| Dosage Suggestions for Hot Flashes | | |
|---|---|---|
| **NUTRIENT OR INTERVENTION** | **TYPICAL DAILY DOSE** | **SUGGESTED PRODUCTS** |
| Black cohosh | 40–80 mg standardized extract | Natural Estrogen with Pomegranate Extract |
| Progesterone | Based on blood test results, symptoms, and physician prescribing | Available by prescription or over the counter |
| Hops extract | 120 mg | Natural Female Support |
| Lignans | 56 mg | |
| Genistein | 25–75 mg | Super-Absorbable Soy Isoflavones, available by prescription |
| Daidzein (Not to be used in conjunction with BHRT, i.e., Bi-Est and Tri-Est formulations) | 20–50 mg | |
| Bioidentical hormone replacement (Natural estrogen, progesterone, and testosterone prescribed to provide individual dosing based on blood test results) | Based on individual blood test results | Available by prescription |

Please know that in the presence of estrogen, progesterone, and testosterone imbalances, it may be impossible to eliminate hot flashes with nutrients alone. Have your blood tested for estrogens (estradiol and estrone), progesterone, DHEA, and testosterone.

## PAINFUL, SWOLLEN BREASTS

According to many doctors the antidote is using bioidentical progesterone and rubbing it right on the breasts to get faster relief. Of course, this makes sense because the painful swollen breasts are likely due to you being estrogen dominant, and as we know by now that means you are not making enough progesterone. Birth control pills stimulate the growth of breast tissue and the retention of fluids, both of which contribute to the swelling.

During the years I blindly took birth control pills, I trusted that they were safe. Even though my body got puffy, my breasts got puffy, and my moods got intense, no doctor expressed concern. No doctor had any remedy; it was just 'part of being a woman'. We've come a long way.

Qualified doctors recommend bioidentical progesterone to balance the estrogen and supplementation with a good multivitamin daily that includes zinc, B complex, vitamin E, magnesium, vitamin C, milk thistle, and other herbs that detoxify the body. Dr. Jonathan Wright also suggests the following herbs: vitex, black cohosh, and dong quai, to help detox and alleviate painful cystic breasts.

### Solutions for Painful, Swollen Breasts

- Double-blind, placebo-controlled trials have indicated that vitex is beneficial for reducing breast pain, menstrual irregularities, and premenstrual complaints.
- Phytoestrogens may be beneficial as well. After two months,

women taking phytoestrogens had less headaches, breast tenderness, cramps, and swelling premenstrually.

| Dosage Suggestions for Painful, Swollen Breasts | | |
|---|---|---|
| **NUTRIENT OR INTERVENTION** | **TYPICAL DAILY DOSE** | **SUGGESTED PRODUCTS** |
| Black cohosh | 40–80 mg standardized extract | Natural Estrogen with Pomegranate Extract |
| Vitex agnus-castus (chasteberry) | 20–40 mg standardized extract | |
| Progesterone | Based on blood test results, symptoms, and physician prescribing | Available by prescription or over the counter |
| Phytoestrogens | 270 mg standardized to contain 40% isoflavones | Super Absorbable Soy Isoflavones |
| High-potency, comprehensive multivitamin | Per label instructions | Life Extension Mix or Two-Per-Day |

# UNEXPLAINED WEIGHT GAIN

If unexplained weight gain is your issue then it's time for you to have a comprehensive weight loss blood test panel to determine your hormone levels and start rebalancing. After you obtain your blood test results, I cannot stress this enough, you must go to a qualified bioidentical hormone replacement (BHRT) doctor. To go to a doctor who has not chosen to specialize in bioidentical hormone replacement is like going to a plumber for a heart transplant; it's often that far out of their area of expertise.

Also, there are many different nutrients to help support a

healthy weight, that are especially effective when combined with proper hormone restoration, diet, and exercise. A big one we are hearing a lot about is the wonderful green coffee extract. While this extract has been working wonders alone, the best approach for weight loss is targeting multiple mechanisms involved in weight loss, from controlling blood sugar levels to preventing absorption of calories.

## Solutions for Weight Gain

- Green coffee extract has been all over the news lately, and with good reason. It targets weight loss through multiple mechanisms. Its strong dual effects of reducing after-meal glucose and inducing meaningful weight loss make it a supplement that virtually every aging person should take *before* eating. Also, it inhibits a special enzyme that is involved in the creation of glucose by the liver. If you want to lose weight you certainly don't want your liver making more glucose!

- A soluble fiber is important to bind to bile acids in our intestine, thus helping to impede absorption of dietary fats. A specially processed propolmannan is a plant-derived fiber that is patented in 33 countries as a purified fiber that does not break down in the digestive tract. Research reveals propolmannan's ability to reduce the rate of carbohydrate absorption and glucose spikes in the blood, both very good things!

- White kidney bean extract contains an inhibitor of amylase (i.e., a pancreatic digestive enzyme required for the conversion of starches to simpler sugars in animals). By inhibiting this enzyme you can help reduce the absorption of high glycemic carbohydrates from starchy foods like potatoes.

- African mango extract, otherwise known as Irvingia, has been shown to reduce fat stores while also helping to support healthy glucose levels. In addition, this West African fruit can help more leptin get into your brain. This effect is important because leptin tells our brains we have eaten enough! If that wasn't sufficient, it also interferes with a special enzyme that converts starch and sugar into stored fat.

- Tryptophan is an essential amino acid and a precursor to serotonin, a powerful neurotransmitter involved in mood and food cravings, especially carbohydrates. Increases in brain levels of serotonin signal that you are full, while decreases signal the desire to eat. Multiple studies have shown that calorie-restricted diets, while successful at reducing weight, also reduce circulating tryptophan levels. This may lead to reduced serotonin synthesis, increased hunger, and a reduction in the probability of maintaining weight loss.

- Often find yourself snacking between meals? Can't help reaching for that extra cookie? Having difficulty exercising portion control? Saffron extract may be just the answer you need. Saffron is a spice that was prized in ancient Persia as a way to enhance mood and relieve stress. Previously available only in Europe, a special standardized saffron extract provides support for healthy body weight by targeting some of the emotional factors that make you eat more when you're trying to eat less. In a clinical study, subjects experienced a greater sense of control over between-meal snacking and a change in eating behavior, without that "jittery feeling" or other undesirable effects. They also reported feeling better about themselves and better in general.

- 7-keto DHEA is a special metabolite of DHEA. Studies have

shown many health benefits of this unique metabolite, but a very important one is weight loss. It helps up-regulate three key thermogenic enzymes in the liver that burn fat. It also is associated with a potential increase in thyroid hormone. These effects result in an increase in resting metabolic rate, which basically means burning more fat, even at rest!

- Green tea polyphenols also help boost resting metabolic rate and help impede the lipase enzyme used to facilitate dietary fat breakdown. This effect results in less fat being absorbed.

- For best results with weight loss you should have your blood tested to get your hormones balanced, identify a healthy diet and exercise program you can stick with, and supplement with nutrients that target different mechanisms of weight loss.

| Dosage Suggestions for Unexplained Weight Gain | | |
|---|---|---|
| NUTRIENT OR INTERVENTION | TYPICAL DAILY DOSE | SUGGESTED PRODUCTS |
| Green coffee extract | 350 mg with each meal | |
| White kidney bean extract | 445 mg before carbohydrate containing meals | Calorie Control Weight Management Formula with CoffeeGenic |
| Propolmannan fiber extract | Follow label instructions | |
| African mango extract | 150 mg with each meal | |
| Green tea extract | 150 mg with each meal | |

| Tryptophan | 500–1,500 mg | Optimized Tryptophan |
| Saffron extract | 88–176 mg | Optimized Saffron with Satiereal® |
| 7-keto DHEA | 100 mg twice a day | 7-Keto DHEA |

## YEAST INFECTIONS AND OVERGROWTH

Yeast interferes with your GI tract. Yeast mycotoxins and bacterial endotoxins from a dysfunctional gut contribute to thyroid dysfunction, which causes decreased dopamine activity (the pleasure center of your brain) and also suppresses pituitary output of the hormone FSH (follicle-stimulating hormone), which stimulates the ovaries to produce estradiol.

When your hormones are 'off' then most likely your gut is imbalanced, which is why you are bloating, constipated, and gaining weight.

So how do you get rid of it? Of course getting your hormones perfectly balanced will go a long way but your needs are immediate. Here are some other solutions

### Solutions for Yeast Infection and Candida

- ReNew Life (RenewLife.com), a company that belongs to my dear friend Brenda Watson and her husband, has a supplement called CandiGONE that "eats" candida. Start slow with CandiGONE because yeast kill is uncomfortable; gas, bloating, and fatigue result from the die-off. Along with your CandiGONE, Brenda recommends you take a daily packet containing 200 billion colony forming units of probiotics while you are doing a candida kill.
- You could also try a douche with apple cider vinegar

(one to two cups) twice daily diluted in a quart of water instead.

- If neither of the above appeals, try an alkalinizing powder called Bio-Terrain available at the Tahoma Clinic in Washington. Keeping alkaline is very important. Yeast cannot live in an alkaline environment (neither can cancer incidentally). Red meat is acid and should be avoided. I have installed an alkaline water dispenser in my kitchen sink and I drink about 4 glasses a day. I feel this keeps me protected not only from yeast, and as a woman who once had cancer I know the importance of keeping my body alkaline for prevention.

## SIMPLE TEST AT HOME FOR CANDIDA

Did you know you can test for candida at home very easily? When you wake up in the morning, before brushing your teeth or eating, spit (it's not ladylike but it is effective) into a clear glass of water to cover the surface. Observe the water periodically for up to five minutes and look for the following signs:

- Strings coming down from your saliva (like jellyfish tentacles).
- The water becomes cloudy.
- The saliva sinks to the bottom of the glass.

Healthy saliva will float on top of the water. If you have these other signs, then likely you have candida overgrowth.

- If you have too much yeast in your body, avoid sugar and anything with sugar in it. I also avoid wine because of the yeast, and breads and all things white: white flour, white rice, even high-starch vegetables like yams, sweet potatoes, and potatoes until you no longer have yeast. These high-starch vegetables are converted to sugar in your body giving your yeast a "happy meal."

- Probiotics are beneficial against yeast infections and are suggested for women who suffer more than three yeast infections per year. Probiotics work by suppressing the growth of yeast in various parts of the body and by inhibiting its ability to stick to cell surfaces.
- Resveratrol can stop candida from converting into its more infectious form, thus making it ideal as a therapy to fight yeast infections.
- Lactoferrin, a protein found in milk, can inhibit the growth of several types of yeast. It has also been shown to enhance the activity of some common antifungal drugs.
- Garlic contains compounds that have been shown to potently inhibit the growth of yeast and fight yeast infections.
- Boric acid can inhibit the growth and reproduction of fungi and can be used intravaginally to treat yeast infections. Boric acid appears to be a safe, effective, and relatively cheap treatment for recurrent yeast infections.

| Dosage Suggestions for Yeast Infections and Overgrowth | | |
| --- | --- | --- |
| NUTRIENT OR INTERVENTION | TYPICAL DAILY DOSE | SUGGESTED PRODUCTS |
| Probiotics | Per label instructions | *Bifido* GI Balance or Theralac |
| Trans-resveratrol | 250 mg | Optimized Resveratrol with Synergistic Grape-Berry Actives |

| Apolactoferrin | 285 mg | Lactoferrin (apolac-toferrin) Caps |
|---|---|---|
| Garlic | 1,200–4,800 mg standardized extract | Optimized Garlic |
| Boric acid suppository | Per label instructions | Available by pre-scription or over the counter |
| High-potency, comprehensive multivitamin | Per label instructions | Life Extension Mix or Two-Per-Day |
| Herbal blend | 2–4 capsules a day | CandiGONE |

## WHERE TO FIND RECOMMENDED SUPPLEMENTS AND REMEDIES

Most of the nutrients, remedies, and recommended tests suggested within these pages can be obtained easily from Life Extension, an organization dedicated to rigorous medical science. You can reach them by calling 1-888-718-5433 or logging on to www.lef.org/goodhealth.

# FINDING A DOCTOR

## FOREVER HEALTH—CONNECTING PATIENTS WITH QUALIFIED PHYSICIANS

In the past, I have provided specific names and contacts to qualified doctors in the resource section at the back of my books. My passion is cutting-edge health, new medicine, and age-management. I practice it, I write about it, and I totally believe in it. My millions of readers are seeking information on how to achieve this lifestyle. They want what I have—robust health with a functional brain, strong healthy bones, balanced hormones, and the energy of someone half my age.

After interviewing many doctors and scientists for my books, I know the solution lies with caring, committed physicians who want to provide the finest health care possible, however, up until now creating a network where doctors and patients can connect has been a challenge. *Every woman and man in our country deserves the option of having access to cutting-edge, quality of life treatments.*

So I am thrilled to share with you information about Forever

Health. Forever Health provides a reliable resource for patients to find qualified physicians in their area. I am proud to be their spokesperson.

In my books, I try to expose my readers to advancements in the world of preventive medicine. I believe in restoration rather than deterioration. I believe we can build our immune system to avoid disease rather than the conventional method of only treating the symptoms of illness.

Forever Health doctors believe as I do. They specialize in age-management, including preventative medicine, bioidentical hormone replacement therapy, vitamins and supplements, and overall health and longevity. I feel confident sending my readers to Forever Health, that they will be able to find qualified physicians in this field of medicine, physicians I would see myself.

The service of finding the right doctor through the Forever Health network is free of charge to the potential patient/reader. To access this incredible service, go to ForeverHealth.com.

# GETTING TESTED

Life Extension has made a special offer to my readers to give you affordable access to proper blood testing and interpretation. Comprehensive blood tests from commercial laboratories can be quite costly, but I have arranged for my readers to obtain special low prices. The good news is you can order these tests yourself and have your blood drawn in a blood drawing station near you at your convenience.

## HORMONE BLOOD TESTS
## AT ULTRA-LOW PRICES

Commercial laboratories, as I just stated, often charge excessive prices for comprehensive hormone testing. I find it far more efficient and cost effective to utilize the blood testing service offered by Life Extension. They offer a special Female Hormone Test Panel that checks:

DHEA
TSH (thyroid-stimulating hormone)

Estradiol (the dominant estrogen)
Progesterone
Free testosterone
CBC and chemistry that includes:
   Total cholesterol
   Glucose
   LDL (bad cholesterol)
   Liver function
   HDL (good cholesterol)
   Kidney function
   Triglycerides
   Red cell count
   Calcium
   Immune cells

The price for all these tests is $149, a fraction of what you'd pay elsewhere. Life Extension will send requisitions and then interpret the results for you afterwards. You can order the Female Hormone Test Panel by calling Life Extension at 1-888-718-5433 or logging on to lef.org/goodhealth. They'll send you a prepaid blood test requisition along with a list of blood draw stations in your area that you can walk into without an appointment.

As a special offer to my readers, Life Extension is offering a *free* six-month membership to anyone who orders the Female Hormone Test Panel. Membership benefits include the monthly *Life Extension Magazine*, along with toll-free phone and e-mail access to knowledgeable health advisors.

Comprehensive blood testing is the critical *first* step to restoring youthful health.

# HYDROCHLORIC ACID DEFICIENCIES

To test for hydrochloric acid deficiencies (an important component to digestion and gut health) you can test with: The Heidelberg PH diagnostic test, although this test must be done under a doctor's supervision.

Meridian Valley Labs tests for hormones, allergies, and blood viscosity. Go to http://meridianvalleylab.com/.

# TESTING FOR FOOD ALLERGIES
## AND FOOD SENSITIVITIES

Most alternative doctors agree the best way to approach testing foods is to first address the two main causes of food reactions. As discussed earlier, one is when your immune system reacts to food via IgE antibodies. This is a true allergy and is fast acting; usually symptoms appear within a few minutes to one to two hours. An example of this type of immune response is when someone has a peanut or shellfish allergy.

The second common way the immune system can respond to food is through a different antibody called IgG. This type of reaction causes a wide range of symptoms that can appear within a few hours to twenty-four to forty-eight hours after eating a food, which makes them much harder to detect since the association with food is harder to figure out. Thus a good approach is to test for both IgE and IgG reactions. A person's immune system can react to a food in both ways or just one of the ways.

For testing for true allergies (IgE) the most common foods that cause problems are:

Beef
Chocolate

Corn

Egg (whole)

Fish/shellfish

Milk (Cow)

Peanut

Pork

Soybean

Wheat

These IgE allergy tests are bundled into a blood panel called Allergen Profile Basic II that my readers can obtain for a special price of $115. There are also specific panels for milk/cheese, grains, fruits, fish/shellfish, etc., for those who want to get even more targeted testing done for certain food groups.

For IgG testing for delayed food reactions there are many more foods that can cause problems. Thus the panel for this type of testing includes 95 common foods and my readers can obtain it for $198.

Lastly, if reactions to wheat are suspected a person should also consider getting a celiac disease test called the Celiac Disease Antibody Screen for $99. This looks at yet another way a person could be reacting to wheat. It is crazy but a person could react to wheat in just one of these three ways I discussed or two of the three, or even all three. It all depends on how out of balance your immune system may be at the time of testing.

Bottom line: Get tested so you can start eliminating foods that may be negatively affecting your life. After one to two weeks of eliminating offending foods people typically report wonderful changes in their health.

## Doctors Data Test

Food allergies can also be tested by taking a comprehensive stool analysis (CSA test) to determine gut imbalances, food intolerances, and candida overgrowth. This test determines the extent of inflammation to differentiate between inflammations with potentially life-threatening implications, like inflammatory bowel disease. This test is available from Doctors Data.

## Where to Find Recommended Supplements

Most of the nutrients, remedies, and recommended tests suggested within the pages of this book can be obtained easily from Life Extension, a trusted organization dedicated to rigorous medical science. You can reach them by calling 1-888-718-5433 or logging on to www.lef.org/goodhealth.

# LETTERS FROM WOMEN LIKE YOU

If you are still worrying, concerned, or just not convinced by me and this book that BHRT is the solution for you and your peri-menopausal symptoms, don't just take my word for it. Research and investigate more. Read as much as you can get your hands on. First, though, read this small sampling of the many, many people who have contacted me throughout the years who say that hormone replacement has changed their lives.

The first letter is from Caroline Somers, my daughter-in-law, who I asked to explain why she feels so grateful for having had access to bioidentical hormones early in life, just as she entered perimenopause.

## CAROLINE'S HORMONE STORY

At the age of thirty-seven I had mastered the fine art of being "superwoman." My husband, Bruce, and I had two beautiful girls, ages six and four. We ran an amaz-ing small business. As co-owners of a successful direct response advertising agency we were producing dozens of commercials for the *LA Times,* DirecTV, Visa, American Airlines, and Hoover to name a few. I had also started working on the side for my mother-in-law, Suzanne, on a little weight loss project called Somersize—a business that exploded into a cottage industry with a series of books, food products, and appliances. In my free time I was overseeing building a new house. Every minute of every day was accounted for, and I was masterfully spinning from one task to the next. The children's birthday parties were spectacular; we were creating successful campaigns for our clients; Suzanne's business was expanding and exciting; our social life was filled with fabulous friends; and the house was a fantasy project.

You can imagine my surprise when I started having hot flashes in what seemed like the prime of my life! Symptoms I was not supposed to even entertain until fifty arrived without warning. Every day started to feel like the worst premenstrual day of my life. Moody! I could whip from weepy to sassy in a mercurial minute. It was an out-of-body experience to hear the shrill voice come out of my mouth, overreacting to something I would have handled deftly in the past.

Fortunately, I had been seeing an antiaging doctor since I was twenty-six years old. Dr. David Allen in Santa Monica understood the importance of bioidentical hormones and could see that I had blunted my hormone production from my high-stress "I can do it all" lifestyle. He had previously done hormone panels on me, so he had a baseline of my hormone levels when all was well. Yes, that's why you need to have a hormone panel done way before you think you are ever in need of it! It was clear that I had dipped below my baseline, when I was feeling at peak performance, and I wanted to get back to that happy, healthy place.

I was also fortunate to have the ultimate hormone-maven as my mother-in-law, and there is no one better to speak with than Suzanne about her very favorite topic—HORMONES!!! She explained that even though I was only thirty-seven, I had likely begun perimenopause, which starts as early as thirteen years before menopause. She went on to explain that this phase can be a little harder to balance because of the drops and surges of your sex hormones—just another way women must learn to adapt to unpredictable situations. But you can either figure it out or . . . become miserable, undesirable, overweight, and a downright bitch? The choice was easy.

Dr. Allen prescribed a bioidentical hormone cocktail of estrogen, progesterone, DHEA, and pregnenolone—along with the normal regime of supplements I had been taking according to deficiencies seen in my blood work. With the first bit of estrogen, I felt better immediately. And then within a couple of months, as my overall levels balanced out, the remainder of my symptoms were relieved and I felt like myself again! I had my fire back; my wit, my sense of humor, my drive, my normal weight.

If you still doubt this is the path for you, you will likely remain a little bitter, a little overweight, and suffer in silence (or loud rage, as is usually the case!). And you also could be at risk for numerous health-related issues caused by loss of hormones.

I have a strong line of female cancers in my family. My maternal grandmother died of ovarian cancer. My mother died of breast cancer. My maternal aunt died of ovarian cancer. People ask me, "Aren't you afraid of taking hormones with all that cancer in your family?" Afraid? Hell, no. I know these bioidentical hormones are protecting me from the diseases of aging because they are keeping my body at its prime. I know the supplements and hormones I take have made my immune system stronger than any cancer cells that may be in my body. I know it because I'm lucky to be with a doctor who thinks outside of the box. I know it from the research Suzanne has exposed me to, and I know it because I have the vitality and energy of a healthy, youthful person.

This year I will celebrate my forty-eighth birthday. That's how old my mother was when she passed away. I used to wonder if I would ever live past forty-eight. Would I leave behind my children as she did? No, I will not repeat the tragic, clipped ending of her life, leaving behind a husband and six kids. I have the information she didn't. I have the resources she didn't. I am proactive about my health. I have access to the doctors who understand how to prevent illness rather than treat the symptoms with drugs that do nothing to eliminate the root of the problem.

It's not my job to tell anyone else what to do or how to live her life, but once you see the benefits, it's hard to imagine you wouldn't want the same thing. I will never experience the symptoms of menopause! From now on, I will continue to adjust my levels to make sure I am healthy and strong and feeling great. WOW! Talk about taking control of the situation. I feel very blessed to be privy to this type of medicine, and extraordinarily blessed to have Suzanne as my earth mother to continue to guide me in the direction of health and wellness.

Caroline's story should be encouraging to you. I witness her balance and happiness on a regular basis. It gives me such pleasure that by embracing her symptoms early on she has been able to enjoy superb life quality.

Here are more voices, like hers. Like yours.

Like many other women I started suffering the effects of perimenopause. Night sweats, hot flashes, itchy dry skin, but worst of all absolutely no sex drive. I had one doctor tell me to drink a glass of wine. (Like that was going to help.) I went to several doctors about having no sex drive, but no one could help me. I read your book and researched and found a compounding pharmacy near me and a doctor that would prescribe them to me. It changed my life. I feel like a teenager again. I lost 40 pounds, as well, that I had struggled with before taking the hormones. I preach to every woman that will listen about the benefits. Thank you for changing my life.

—Myrna S.

I am forty-eight years old and currently using BHRT. I have an active life. I have three boys who are fifteen, thirteen, and ten. My husband owns a successful food distribution company. One day runs into another. I am cook, laundry person, money manager, educational advocate, and I am sure I can come up with many more titles. I have read your books and have seen you on different shows talking about BHRT. At first I took in the information and stored it away, because I thought I was not experiencing any symptoms and did not think it applied to me. Well, was I wrong! I was feeling like I had the flu or was about to get it. I was tired all the time, which didn't make sense because I worked out, ate healthy, and slept well. More symptoms started popping up. I was feeling overwhelmed, depressed, crying in the middle of the day while folding clothes. I could not even decide what to make my family for dinner. I knew I had to do something. After finding out my estrogen and progesterone were low I started the process of balancing out my system. The estrogen made a huge difference. I am quite sensitive to hormone fluctuations, so I work with my doctor still. But it is so worth it. I take estradiol, progesterone, and a little testosterone. I am able to function again and take care of all my boys.

—Gretchen B.

I began taking bioidentical hormones in March 2012. Prior to this I knew something wasn't right but trying to get a doctor (the right kind of doctor) to listen to you is very hard. Thankfully I now have the right doctor. I was anxious, not sleeping well, no sex drive, among a few other things. I feel like a new person. I noticed immediate results. My anxiousness and sleep issues were solved right away. I am very thankful for your book and my doctor suggesting I read it. It got my doctor and me talking and got me to take a more proactive approach to my health.

—Sue T.

I am a busy wife of an MLB executive. I do charity work and travel a lot. I tried to ignore heavy bleeding for three out of five days of my cycle for several years. I found myself scheduling trips around my cycle out of fear that I would be on a flight and not able to get up every ten to fifteen minutes to use the lavatory. There was an embarrassing time when we were guests for dinner at another baseball executive's home and I was in the bathroom repeatedly. My husband and I ended up having to leave the dinner early because I ran out of sanitary pads, and the hostess had already given me everything she had. I was miserable. By the time we were leaving, I realized that I had soiled my slacks and may have even soiled the suede chair in the dining room where we ate. By the time we arrived home, it was a mess; I was a mess. The years of heavy bleeding caused me to become anemic and always tired. Now, I read everything I can that you write because you research everything and understand what women need to know to be informed. I call it cutting to the chase. Thank you, Suzanne Somers, for all your hard work and research, and for writing this book.

—Linda S.

I was about to lose my mind. I was tired and absent-minded and cried all of the time. I went to see a neurologist and an endocrinologist, and they both told me I was just getting older and I needed to see a psychiatric doctor to help with the crying. I called a friend who was a doctor for advice. He told me to go straight to a lab and do blood work. Then I went to get your books. What a lifesaver you both have been to me.

—Lisa A.

I started perimenopause symptoms when I was forty-four. I suffered mood swings, night sweats, day sweats, lack of sexual drive, and weight gain for four years. I finally could not take it anymore and went to my doctor who prescribed a hormone replacement patch, Climara Pro. It worked very well, took away all the symptoms; except for one problem, dense cystic breasts. I developed benign tumors in both of my breasts. Two surgeries later, I decided to go cold turkey and stop using the patch from fear of developing breast cancer. I went with no hormone replacement for three years. I had full-blown menopause, it came back with a vengeance worse than before. I knew about Suzanne's books, being an avid reader I often went to Barnes and Noble, and I had read excerpts from *Ageless*. At first I was skeptical but a friend of mine who had read the book, referred me to a local doctor. Dr. Tara Solomon changed my life. After blood work and a lengthy consultation she prescribed bioidentical hormone replacement. BHRT has changed my life. In two weeks I was a fully functioning, sexy woman again. My husband of thirty-four years is very happy and thankful. I have been on BHRT for two years. I have had clean mammograms and ultrasounds for two years. No lumpy breasts. No side effects of any kind with the exception of a very elevated libido (no complaint from my husband). I recommend it to all the women suffering from menopause. And the cost is minimal. This is my story. I am fifty-six years old and loving life. Thank you.

—Maggie A.

Before I started on hormones I had a very low sex drive and lots of vaginal dryness. I got better with the dryness using estrogen and progesterone, but when I started using low doses of testosterone. . . . WOW, did my desire for sex explode. I try not to take too much testosterone, as I can see why it can be abused. It makes you feel so vibrant and strong. I take what I am supposed to and if my blood tests show that I am high I will stop it for a while. Sadly, if I stop for too long my libido tanks fast. So I try now to stay on top of it and stick to what my doctor tells me. I feel I would have no sex drive at all if not for my replacement hormones.

—Kelly L.

I started on bioidentical hormones years ago when I first read about them in your books and my relationship with my husband, who is also on them, is better and sexier than ever . . . EVER! It wasn't that way before BHRT. We slept together, but rarely were intimate. Yes, we hugged and kissed in bed, but nothing serious. We love our sex life together now and giggle a lot every time we conclude a couple of hours of lovemaking. My husband claims that were it not for you, we would be hobbling along and missing all the fun. Since BHRT, my face is less wrinkled, my muscle tone is firm, my skin is smooth and tight.

You have changed my life.

You have saved my life.

You have saved my marriage.

You have gifted me with an incredible quality of life.

You have given me good reason to work on my health and break through that one hundred mark and celebrate by having sex with my husband.

Thank you, thank you, thank you.

—Marge

I was forty-eight when I had my first appointment with the doctor in our area that uses bioidentical hormones. I am perimenopausal and still have fairly regular periods. However, I had gained fifteen pounds over the past few years, had a lower libido, was irritable, and had dry skin and achy joints. After my "hormone" doctor reviewed my blood work she put me on Armor thyroid to boost my thyroid level, and progesterone for fourteen days of my cycle, plus I began testosterone and estrogen. I saw a difference in just over two weeks! Dry skin gone, libido up, aches gone! I lost twenty pounds after four months of using the bioidentical hormones. This was three years ago. Unfortunately my insurance won't cover it because it doesn't recognize bioidenticals as a proven treatment therapy. Hopefully, this will change. I am blond and fair and I have noticed an increased amount of facial hair—so now waxing my chin and lip area is part of my regime. I am told this is a common side effect for some of us.

The bioidentical treatments I get are pricey, but make such a difference in how I feel and give me a calmer sense of well-being because my hormones are more balanced. Bioidenticals have really helped me feel more energetic and youthful! I like to think that when we begin to feel good and beautiful on the inside it can't help but radiate to our outer self—a bonus!"

—Cindy B.

I was on our bucket list vacation with my husband when my hot flashes and insomnia became so unpleasant that I decided to see a doctor as soon as I returned home.

I was put on a prescription for synthetic hormones that made me so miserable I considered taking my own life. My family was afraid to leave me alone. I stayed in bed day after day trying to avoid human contact. I had become a monster. I hated everyone including myself. I later learned that I was experiencing something called "roid rage." After several months of this awful existence, I made an appointment at a natural medical clinic to inquire about my options. I was able to wean off the synthetic hormones and start bioidentical hormones and I am a new woman. I feel wonderful and whole again. I am grateful for every day of my life. The added bonus is that my sex drive has returned after being nonexistent for years. I never thought that would happen! That was

three years ago. My health is still good. I still feel attrac-
tive and empowered.

—Shannon H.

It's not a "suddenly wake up and feel awful" feeling. It's
not overnight. It is a slow gradual decline down a spiral
staircase. And then one day, you realize how low you've
descended. You can't sleep a full night anymore. You are
cranky every day, and for no reason. Your hairbrush is
full of hair and you wonder why you're not bald yet. You
get unbearably hot in front of an air conditioner. You forget important details. You can't tolerate your husband's
touch. You can't seem to ever get enough lotion on your
dry skin. And the scale rises, it seems, daily. Clothes become tighter until you aren't wearing more than half your
wardrobe. It's a cruel joke.

I was desperate to help myself (and my poor family) to stop this ruthless decay. Once I started a tailored
program for bioidentical hormone replacement therapy,
I began to feel normal again. No, no. That's not right. I
didn't just feel normal. I felt vital. I felt better than I had in
years. My skin became soft, my hair stopped falling out. I
started smiling and laughing again. Nothing bothered me
anymore. I desired my husband more than I had when we
were young! My memory returned. No more night sweats.
The hot flashes vanished.

—Shannon S.

In 2007, at age forty-nine, I suddenly had no energy. I had
read a lot about bioidentical hormones and had already
been using progesterone cream for about eight years (to
prevent breast cancer by balancing my hormones), so I

decided to start using estriol and testosterone creams. Almost immediately, I had much more energy and at a time in my life when I was dealing with my daughter's health crisis, I needed it. I am fifty-four now, still using the hormones, and I sailed through menopause with the only symptom or side effect being my cessation of menses: no hot flashes, no mood swings. I feel great. A couple of years ago my husband added testosterone shots to his health regimen, and together with mine that makes for an incredible sex life in our midfifties. Who would have dreamed it!

—Jackie D.

# FURTHER READING

Blaylock, Russell L., MD. *Excitotoxins: The Taste That Kills*. Royal Oak, Mich.: Health Press, 1996.

Campbell, T. Colin, PhD, and Thomas M. Campbell II, MD. *The China Study: The Most Comprehensive Study of Nutrition Ever Conducted and the Startling Implications for Diet, Weight Loss and Long-Term Health*. Dallas, Tex.: BenBella Books, 2006.

Cloutier, Pierre, MD. *Optimal Physiology for Life*. Melbourne, Fla.: Blue Note Books, 2012.

Dach, Jeffrey, MD. *Bioidentical Hormones 101*. iUniverse, 2011.

Hertoghe, Thierry, MD. *The Hormone Solution: Stay Younger Longer with Natural Hormone and Nutrition Therapies*. New York: Three Rivers Press, 2002.

Hoffman, Ronald L., MD. *Tired All the Time: How to Regain Your Lost Energy*. New York: Gallery Books, 1996.

Kekich, David A. *Life Extension Express*. BookSurge.com, 2009.

Lee, John R., MD, and Virginia Hopkins. *Dr. John Lee's Hormone Balance Made Simple: The Essential How-To Guide to Symptoms, Dosage, Timing and More*. New York: Grand Central Life & Style, 2006.

Miller, Philip Lee, MD, and the Life Extension Foundation. *The Life Extension Revolution: The New Science of Growing Older Without Aging*. New York: Bantam Books, 2005.

Norling, Sharon, MD. *Your Doctor Is Wrong*. CreateSpace, 2012.

Pelton, Ross, R.Ph., CCN. *The Pill Problem: How to Protect Your Health from the Side Effects of Oral Contraceptives*, 2013.

Rogers, Sherry A., MD. *Detoxify or Die*. Hampton, Va.: Prestige, 2002.

Rothenberg, Ron, MD, Kathleen Becker, and Kris Hart. *Forever Ageless*. Encinitas, Calif.: HealthSpan Institute, 2007.

Shoemaker, Ritchie, MD. *Surviving Mold*. Otter Bay Books, 2010.

Shulman, Neil, MD, Jack Birge, MD, and Joon Ahn, MD. *Your Body's Red Light Warning Signals*. New York: Delta, 2009.

Simpson, Kathryn R., MS, and Thierry Hertoghe, MD. *The Women's Guide to Thyroid Health: Comprehensive Solutions for All Your Thyroid Symptoms*. Oakland, Calif.: New Harbinger, 2009.

Somers, Suzanne. *Ageless: The Naked Truth About Bioidentical Hormones*. New York: Three Rivers Press, 2007.

———*Breakthrough: Eight Steps to Wellness*. New York: Three Rivers Press, 2009.

———*The Sexy Years: Discover the Hormone Connection*. New York: Three Rivers Press, 2005.

Watson, Brenda, CNC. *The Road to Perfect Health—How Probiotics Balance Your Gut and Heal Your Body*. Sherman Oaks, Calif.: Health Point Press, 2011.

## Studies That Show the Safety and Efficacy of BHRT

As you have read in this book, there is considerable misinformation as to the safety of hormone replacement. Clearly, as has been established in this book, those safety concerns are about synthetic fake hormone replacement. This can be verified by reading the Women's Health Initiative (visit www.nhlbi.nih.gov).

I wanted to share a few other studies and papers on the efficacy, safety, and health-restoring benefits of replacing hormones correctly with BHRT.

Dach, Jeffrey, MD. "Hormone Replacement Therapy HRT Does NOT Cause Breast Cancer, New Study," *Jeffrey Dach MD Bioidentical Hormone Blog*, posted March 16, 2012.

Faloon, William. "The Unscientific Bioidentical Hormone Debate," *Life Extension Magazine*, October 2009.

Life Extension Foundation. "Bioidentical Hormones: Why Are They Still Controversial," *Life Extension Magazine*, October 2009.

Moskowitz, Deborah, MD. "A Comprehensive Review of the Safety and Efficacy of Bioidentical Hormones," *American College for Advancement in Medicine IM Blog*, August 12, 2011.

Ruiz, Andres D., Kelly R. Daniels, Jamie C. Barner et al. "Effectiveness of Compounded Bioidentical Hormone Replacement Therapy: An Observational Cohort Study," *BMC Women's Health* 11 (2011): 27.

## Additional Studies

Bakken, K., A. Fournier, E. Lund et al. "Menopausal Hormone Therapy and Breast Cancer Risk: Impact of Different Treatments: The European Prospective Investigation into Cancer and Nutrition," *International Journal of Cancer* 128, no. 1 (January 2011): 144–156.

Batur, P., C. E. Blixen, H. C. Moore et al. "Menopausal Hormone Therapy (HT) in Patients with Breast Cancer," *Maturitas* 53, no. 2 (January 20, 2006) 123–132.

Beral, V., and Million Women Study Collaborators. "Breast Cancer and Hormone-Replacement Therapy in the Million Women Study," *Lancet* 362, no. 9382 (August 9, 2003): 419–427.

Brooke, D. G., E. J. Shelley, C. G. Roberts et al. "Synthesis and In Vitro Evaluation of Analogues of Avocado-Produced Toxin (+)-(R)-persin in Human Breast Cancer Cells," *Bioorganic and Medicinal Chemistry* 19, no. 23 (December 1, 2011): 7033–7043.

Chlebowski, Rowan T., MD, PhD; Susan L. Hendrix, DO; Robert D. Langer, MD, MPH et al. "Cancer and Mammography in Healthy Postmenopausal Women," *Journal of the American Medical Association* 289, no. 24 (June 25, 2003): 3243–3253.

Christante, D., S. Pommier, J. Garreau et al. "Improved Breast Cancer Survival Among Hormone Replacement Therapy Users Is Durable After 5 Years of Additional Follow-Up," *American Journal of Surgery* 196, no. 4 (October 2008): 505–511.

Clemente, C., F. Russo, M. G. Caruso et al. "Ceruloplasmin Serum Level in Post-Menopausal Women Treated with Oral Estrogens Administered at Different Times," *Hormone and Metabolic Research* 24, no. 4 (April 1992): 191–193.

De Leo, M., R. Pibonello, R. S. Auriemma et al. "Cardiovascular Disease in Cushing's Syndrome: Heart Versus Vasculature," *Neuroendocrinology* 92, supp. 1 (2010): 50–54.

Dew, J. E., B. G. Wren, and J. A. Eden. "Tamoxifen, Hormone Receptors and Hormone Replacement Therapy in Women Previously Treated for Breast Cancer: A Cohort Study," *Climacteric* 5, no. 2 (June 2002): 151–155.

Durna, E. M., G. Z. Heller, L. R. Leader et al. "Breast Cancer in Premenopausal Women: Recurrence and Survival Rates and Relationship to Hormone Replacement Therapy," *Climacteric* 7, no. 3 (September 2004): 284–291.

Espié, M., J. P. Daures, T. Chevallier et al. "Breast Cancer Incidence and Hormone Replacement Therapy: Results from the MISSION Study, Prospective Phase," *Gynecological Endocrinology* 23, no. 7 (July 2007): 391–397.

Fournier, A., F. Berrino, and F. Clavel-Chapelon. "Unequal Risks for Breast Cancer Associated with Different Hormone Replacement Therapies: Results from the E3N Cohort Study," *Breast Cancer Research and Treatment* 107, no. 1 (January 2008): 103–111.

Hadhazy, Adam. "Think Twice: How the Gut's 'Second Brain' Influences Mood and Well-Being," scientificamerican.com (February 12, 2010). www.scientificamerican.com/article.cfm?id=gut-second-brain.

Ives, Jeffrey C., PhD; Mark Alderman, MS, ATC; and Susan E. Stred, MD. "Hypopituitarism After Multiple Concussions: A Retrospective Case Study in an Adolescent Male," *Journal of Athletic Training* 42, no. 3 (July–Sept. 2007): 431–439.

Jick, H., A. M. Walker, and K. J. Rothman. "The Epidemic of Endometrial Cancer: A Commentary," *American Journal of Public Health* 70, no. 3 (March 1980): 264–267.

Mason, G. A., C. H. Walker, and A. J. Prange Jr. "L-triiodothyronine: Is This Peripheral Hormone a Central Neurotransmitter?" *Neuropsychopharmacology* 8, no. 3 (May 1993): 253–258.

McCarthy, M. M. "Estrogen Modulation of Oxytocin and Its Relation to Behavior," *Advances in Experimental Medicine and Biology* 395 (1995): 235–245.

Menna, M. Abdel-Dayem, and Mohamed S. Elgendy. "Effects of Chronic Estradiol Treatment on the Thyroid Gland Structure and Function of Ovariectomized Rats," *BMC Research Notes,* published online (August 30, 2009). www.biomedicalcentral.com/1756-0500/2/173.

Meyers, David G., Daniel Strickland, Pierre A. Maloley et al. "Possible Association of a Reduction in Cardiovascular Events with Blood Donation," *Heart* 78 (1997): 188–193.

Persson, Ingemar, Jonathan Yuen, Leif Bergkvist et al. "Cancer Incidence and Mortality in Women Receiving Estrogen and Estrogen-Progestin Replacement Therapy—Long-Term Follow-up of a Swedish Cohort," *International Journal of Cancer* 67, no. 3 (July 29, 1996): 327–332.

Rossouw, J. E., G. L. Anderson, R. L. Prentice et al. "Risks and Benefits of Estrogen Plus Progestin in Healthy Postmenopausal Women: Principal Results from the Women's Health Initiative Randomized Controlled Trial," *Journal of the American Medical Association* 288, no. 3 (July 17, 2002): 321–323. For more information about the Women's Health Initiative, visit www.nhlbi.nih.gov.

Saeki, Toshiaki, Muneo Sano, Yoshifumi Komoike et al. "No Increase of Breast Cancer Incidence in Japanese Women Who Received Hormone Replacement Therapy: Overview of a Case-Control Study of Breast Cancer Risk in Japan," *International Journal of Clinical Oncology* 13, no. 1 (February 2008): 8–11.

Salonen, Jukka T., Tomi-Pekka Tuomainen, Riitta Salonen et al. "Donation of Blood Is Associated with Reduced Risk of Myocardial Infarction," *American Journal of Epidemiology* 148, no. 5 (1998): 445–451.

Schairer, C., H. O. Adami, R. Hoover, and I. Persson. "Cause-Specific Mortality in Women Receiving Hormone Replacement Therapy," *Epidemiology* 8, no. 1 (January 1997): 59–65.

Schairer, C., J. Lubin, R. Troisi et al. "Menopausal Estrogen and Estrogen-Progestin Replacement Therapy and Breast Cancer Risk," *Journal of the American Medical Association* 283, no. 4, (January 26, 2000): 485–491.

Sintzel, F., M. Mallaret, T. Bougerol. "Potentializing of Tricyclics and Serotoninergics by Thyroid Hormones in Resistant Depressive Disorders," *Encephale* 30, no. 3 (May–June 2004): 267–275.

University of Maryland Medical Center. "Dehydroepiandrosterone," www.umm.edu (April 7, 2011). www.umm.edu/altmed/articles/dehydroepiandrosterone-000299.htm.

Vighi, G., F. Marcucci, L. Sensi, G. Di Cara, and F. Frati. "Allergy and the Gastrointestinal System," *Clinical and Experimental Immunology* 153, supp. 1 (September 2008): 3–6.

Vongpatanasin W., M. Tuncel, Z. Wang et al. "Differential Effects of Oral Versus Transdermal Estrogen Replacement Therapy on C-Reactive Protein in Postmenopausal Women," *Journal of the American College of Cardiology* 41, no. 8 (April 2003): 1358–1363.

Wassertheil-Smoller, Sylvia, PhD; Susan Hendrix, DO; Marian Limacher, MD et al. "Effect of Estrogen Plus Progestin on Stroke in Postmenopausal Women," *Journal of the American Medical Association* 289, no. 20 (May 28, 2003): 2673–2684.

Willis, D. B., E. E. Calle, H. L. Miracle-McMahill, and C. W. Heath Jr. "Estrogen Replacement Therapy and Risk of Fatal Breast Cancer in a Prospective Cohort of Postmenopausal Women in the United States," *Cancer Causes and Control* 7, no. 4 (July 1996): 449–457.

# INDEX

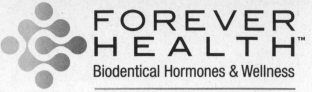
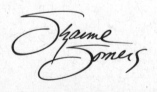